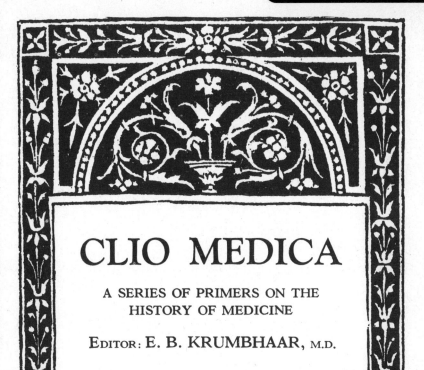

CLIO MEDICA

A SERIES OF PRIMERS ON THE HISTORY OF MEDICINE

EDITOR: E. B. KRUMBHAAR, M.D.

XIX

PATHOLOGY

BY

E. B. KRUMBHAAR, M.D.

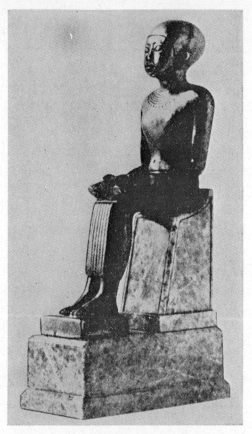

FIG. 1. I-Em-Hotep, the Egyptian God of Medicine.
(From an old Egyptian statuette.)

CLIO MEDICA

PATHOLOGY

BY

E. B. KRUMBHAAR, M.D.

Professor of Pathology
University of Pennsylvania
School of Medicine

WITH 18 ILLUSTRATIONS

HAFNER PUBLISHING COMPANY
NEW YORK
1962

Reprint Edition
by arrangement
1962

Published by
HAFNER PUBLISHING COMPANY, INC.
New York 3, N. Y.

Library of Congress Catalog Card Number: 62-15039

First Edition
© copyright 1937
Paul B. Hoeber, Inc.

Printed in the U.S.A.
_____

NOBLE OFFSET PRINTERS, INC.
NEW YORK 3, N.Y.

To one

who has inspired undertakings and lightened labors with her sought advice and unconscious example.

"The way of thinking of the old art of healing came so near to truth that one should take it more into consideration and wonder at the discoveries made in spite of so great a lack of knowledge." (HIPPOCRATES.)

"Learning without thinking is labour lost,
  Thinking without learning is perilous." (CONFUCIUS.)

"History maketh a young man to be old without either wrinkles or gray hairs; privileging him with the experience of age without either the infirmities or inconveniences thereof. Yea, it not only maketh things past present, but enableth one to make a rational conjecture of things to come." (FULLER.)

"We stand upon the intellectual shoulders of those medical giants of bygone days and, because of the help they afford us, we are able to see a little more clearly than they were able to do." (CLAUDE BERNARD.)

"We cannot know modern medicine unless we study it as a whole, in the past as well as in the present." (CLIFFORD ALLBUTT.)

EDITOR'S PREFACE

THIS little volume is one of a series of handbooks which under the general title of "Clio Medica" aims at presenting in a concise and readable form a number of special phases of the long and complex history that underlies the great edifice of modern medical science.

Since the times of the Aldines and Elzevirs, small easily portable booklets have been popular with the intelligent reader. Today books that add no appreciable burden to the coat pocket are real helps to the busy worker or student in gaining ready access to considerable worth-while reading. Such booklets, too, seem peculiarly appropriate for a new line of approach to such a subject as the History of Medicine from a different point of view than has hitherto maintained. From the very nature of this subject, when treated in a general way, it has thus far appeared either in ponderous tomes or, if in smaller volumes, in such scanty garb that almost no details of the costume are depictable. Then, too, the strictly chronological method of approach, with emphasis on prominent individuals, becomes almost a necessary form of treatment in the comprehensive general histories. The searcher for knowledge of the history of some small branch of the subject—a specialty, let us say, or the progress of medicine in this or that country—is thus forced to hunt, often painfully with help of index and marker, through the pages of the larger book or books, to be rewarded with a necessarily disconnected and usually incomplete presentation.

Our hope is that the series "Clio Medica" will obviate these difficulties. Conveniently small and inexpensive, yet prepared by recognized authorities in their chosen field, each volume aims to present the story of some individualized phase of the history of medicine in such compact, connected, convincing and reasonably complete form that the medical undergraduate, the specialist, the busy general practitioner and the "intelligent layman" will all be attracted to a few hours' reading, which in many cases may prove to be the introduction to an awakened interest to a more comprehensive study.

An increasing interest has recently become manifest in the history of medicine in the English speaking as well as in other countries, as is shown by the successful formation of new societies, journals and institutes for the study of the subject. The times, then, seem auspicious for this venture. Several volumes of the series have already appeared; as others materialize still more will be undertaken, with the possibility of a large number being attained. We bespeak the support of our colleagues and friends and pray that the Goddess whose name we have used to designate our series may deign to foster the undertaking!

E. B. KRUMBHAAR.

PHILADELPHIA, PA.

AUTHOR'S PREFACE

WHEN we consider one of the broader definitions of Pathology—such as "The study of the causes of and the effects (both structural and functional) produced by disease"—we at once realize that a consideration of its history might properly be almost co-terminous with that of medicine. Obviously then, for practical purposes, much that is truly pathological must be omitted from a special history of the subject, and still more from a primer such as the present booklet. And yet we must even more carefully avoid the other extreme, from which the present medical generation is but beginning to emerge, of confusing the larger subject with its subdivision, pathological anatomy. Even though in this series of historical booklets much of etiology and the pathology of the "Specialties" must be left to other volumes on "Bacteriology," "Parasitology" and the respective specialties, nevertheless space must be given here to historical consideration of the nature of disease, as illustrating views of pathologic physiology, even more than to details of changes in structure—important as the latter may have been in the development of medical science.

No apology should be needed for consuming a reader's time that is spent on the history of disease, constituting, as it does, both a highly desirable equipment for even the most practical of men and a pleasant and useful recreation for the broadminded physician. While the function of furnishing facts is a necessary and important preliminary, the arrangement and interpretation of these facts is a more important service of history, which by tracing development, change and readjustment gives us a sound basis for placing ourselves in proper relation to both the present and expected forces, tendencies and problems to which we must adapt ourselves as well as may be. The directions in which knowledge of disease has developed in the past and the methods by which it has extricated itself from error are reliable aids, *mutatis mutandis,* in coping with the medical needs of the present and with the probable tendencies of the future.

In preparing this little book the customary histories of pathology have been consulted and original sources examined as carefully as is compatible with the demands made by an active research and teaching university department; but it must be freely admitted that if it were not for previous reading *per amore,* the intensive historical research that has been specially made for this end would have been quite inadequate. In this connection, acknowledgment is gladly made to Garrison's "History of Medicine" and Long's "History of Pathology"; without the support of these excellent books, the preparation of even this small work would probably not have been undertaken. My thanks are also gratefully extended to W. B. McDaniel, 2d, Librarian of the College of Physicians, for his help in tracing some bibliographic obscurities and in textual criticism; also to Miss M. C. Pfeiffer and Mr. H. Kaplan, medical students who aided in the preparation of the Chronological Table.

In this volume, instead of the customary treatment by strict chronological sequence, the main trends have been treated in separate chapters, with consequent occasional overlapping of dates, that it is hoped will not be enough to be confusing. Thus some eighteenth century theories of disease (really medieval in quality) are considered in an earlier chapter than anatomical concepts that held sway some two or three centuries earlier.

It would have been pleasant to have included in the text references to disease as found in general literature. Shakespeare, of course, gives a number of brilliant thumbnail sketches, as Wainwright has brought out in his "Medical and Surgical Knowledge of William Shakespeare" (New York, 1915); and in Kipling's tales one can find examples of opium poisoning, aphasia, hysteria, hypochondriasis, tabes dorsalis, leprosy and plague and other disease conditions. Also literary characters suffering from consumption and cancer may frequently be found. But how seldom do we find in fiction recognizable depictions of such conditions as floating kidney (as in Tolstoi's Ivan Ilyich) or aphasia (Wilhelm Meister), or even of prenatal influences on the mind (as in Holmes' Elsie Venner) and on the body (as in Malet's Sir Richard Calmady). The discrepancy, compared to the many lesions depicted by artists, as found in our museums of painting and sculpture and described by Eugen Hollander, Veth and others, is indeed striking. Space has forbidden inclusion of this diversion.

Important events in the progress of pathology, interpreted broadly, have been assembled in a chronological list. An attempt to include many "first descriptions" of disease in this list often demanded dogmatic decision as to what constituted a first description. This has sometimes been partly alleviated by inserting other candidates in brackets. As I know of no other similar list, I hope that it may increase the usefulness of this small volume as a book of reference, in addition to whatever qualities its text may possess as instructive reading.

E. B. K.

Philadelphia, Pa.
May, 1937.

CONTENTS

LIST OF ILLUSTRATIONS

CLIO MEDICA

PATHOLOGY

CHAPTER I

PRIMITIVE, CLASSICAL AND MEDIEVAL PATHOLOGIC CONCEPTS. PATHOLOGY OF ANTIQUITY

PREHISTORIC. Disease is known to have existed through many geologic ages. Concepts of the cause and nature of disease necessarily followed long after the earliest beginnings of man's treatment of the sick and wounded; nevertheless we have sufficient evidence, both in the remains of extinct races and in the practices of races still existing in a cultural state equivalent to that of the Prehistoric Era, that often elaborate ideas existed about the nature of disease in extremely early stages of racial development.

From time immemorial, man has seen "God in clouds or hears him in the wind," and it is only to be expected that he would attribute mysterious disease to supernatural agencies. Thus we usually find disease to have been associated with some religious belief, and the witch doctor of the tribe to have cared for both spiritual and

physical ills, whether in the most primitive
stages of human existence or in various successful modern cults. In the commonest form of
primitive culture, diseases are caused by malevo-
lent demons or human enemies. These may be
warded off by the possession of charms or totems,
or by the observance of taboos or by sacrifices,
whose distorted equivalents may still be found
here and there even in the most civilized com-
munities. The remarkable trephines in the skulls
of pre-Columbian Peruvians, like those of some
modern savages, were in all probability designed
to aid the escape of a pain-causing demon rather
than for more rational purposes. Sometimes the
evil influence is looked upon as triumphing by
having projected something harmful into the victim's body or abstracted something from it. This
of course suggests our present concepts of infectious diseases, on the one hand, and deficiency
diseases, on the other. If something necessary has
been abstracted, the attempt may be made to supply the deficiency from the body of the enemy
(cannibalism) or from the totem animal of the
demon enemy. If evil matter has been inserted,
the harmful agency may be combated with appropriate magic or transferred to another—hence,
the scapegoat of the Jews, the φαρμακαι of the
Greeks, and one of the functions attributed by
the Romans to Saturn. Anglo-Saxon belief in the
supernatural quality of disease is shown, too, by
various healing rituals, such as the passage of
a child through a cloven ashtree to cure hernia
(Gilbert White) or through the Holed Stone
of Lanyon, Cornwall, to cure scrofula. Here, as
with the "eye of the needle" tree at Killarney,
which ensures long life and safe delivery to preg-

nant women, belief in the regulative power of
the supernatural is shown thriving far from and
long after its far distant Eastern sources (India?).

Other long-accepted supernatural factors in
the causation of disease, primitive in origin but
surviving into civilized times, are to be found
in the effects of the stars (astrology), the moon
(lunacy or the moon's effect on the mental or
physical state). The mysterious effect of numbers may be traced back through Pythagoras and
the Chaldaeans to beyond the dawn of history.
Certain numbers (different for different races)
often confer health on the newborn or are potent
in curing disease by inference; others are po-
tentially harmful. The persistence of the importance of numbers into modern times (for example, the humoral theory and the critical days
in pneumonia) is still apparent.

Human powers, too, were thought to be able
to produce disease in the body of the savage,
whose whole existence was surrounded by the
mysterious forces of evil. The evil eye, which
must still be warded off in Sicily if bodily harm
is not to follow, has been observed through the
ages and by widespread peoples; though, unfortunately for many sick people, belief in the
equivalent potency of human aid has largely
been lost. Scrofula, for instance, can no longer
be cured by the King's touch, or blindness and
paralysis by an Emperor, a saint or a child
with a caul, though the miracles of Lourdes and
the cures of Christian Science healers continue,
with occasional unexpected support from those
in the high seats of science. The undoubted influence of mind over the diseased body is only

beginning to be understood and properly utilized. Unreasonable and misapplied belief in the healing or ha. ning powers of magic is still, to be sure, widespread: the Hex doctors of Lancaster, Pennsylvania, who committed murder in the cause of magic came to trial in 1929.

While such uncultured views of the causes and nature of disease could be multiplied almost *ad lib*, pathologic anatomy at this stage of civilization was and long remained conspicuous by its absence. Though we may assume that primitive races observed superficial lesions or even the interiors of their friends who had been mutilated by hostile tribes or animals, still we have no indication that their ideas of disease were thereby influenced. That diseases as we know them today existed, however, is amply proved by the paleopathologic studies of Ruffer, Elliot Smith, Moodie and others. From paleozoic times, ages before man existed, reptilian bones bear witness to the existence of necrosis, exostoses, osteomyelitis, arthritis, bony tumors, healing of fractures, carious teeth—in fact, most of the lesions that one would expect to find in bony structures today. The statement has even been hazarded that pathogenic bacteria first appeared in the paleozoic age, and actinomycosis has been reported in a pliocene fossil.

Human pathology has been similarly enriched. Whether we regard the Venus of Willendorf and other steatopygous prehistoric relics as examples of pathologic obesity or of a prehistoric sculptor's idea of beauty, or of both, there can be no question of the existence of many lesions, identical with those of today, in the earliest known human remains. A large exostosis was found on the oldest known human bone—the femur of Pithecanthropus erectus; carious teeth and mandibular abscess appear in the Rhodesian man; the first found Neanderthal man showed a healed fracture of the ulna and signs of rickets in the humerus; a number of Egyptian mummies had arthritis and Pott's disease, and early Egyptian art shows unmistakable achondroplasia and poliomyelitis. When one considers how comparatively few diseases produce bony lesions and the scarcity of the material for study, the great antiquity of disease much as we know it today seems to have firm support.

Sumerian-Assyrian. Just as the most modern researches have shown that the Sumerian (Akkadian-Assyro-Babylonian) civilization can apparently be traced back even further than the Egyptian, so the Code of Hammurabi (2250 B.C.) antedates the earliest existing Egyptian medical writings, though the actual priority of medical knowledge in the two regions is still unsolved, and the question fluctuates with the discoveries from year to year. Our chief knowledge of Assyrian medicine comes from the writings of a much later period, the library of Assurbanipal (668-625 B.C.). From the Hammurabi code and from the early brick inscriptions, we learn that the medical profession was then already far advanced. Abscesses and infected wounds, and their proper surgical treatment, had been recognized. Couching for cataract, another procedure adopted by the Babylonians, is indicative of the superiority of their surgical to medical practice. This latter, as in all the beginnings of medicine, was dominated by the demonic concept of disease, so that the opportunities offered by the frequent examinations of animal viscera by the soothsayers bore little or no fruit. Monsters and abnormally large and small organs were recognized but were only significant as omens. On the other hand, Thompson and Sudhoff show that these peoples had fairly good concepts of gonorrhea, pediculosis, scabies, paralysis, epilepsy and similar diseases. Their appreciation of the transmissibility of leprosy is evidenced by their practice of expelling lepers from the community.

Egypt. I-em-hotep, generally regarded as the first known physician, lived in the third dynasty, before 2900 B.C. He was later elevated to divine rank as the chief god of medicine, but of his human contributions to medicine we know nothing. The ancient Egyptian practice of embalming must have exposed countless lesions of internal organs to the view of the *taricheutes* who eviscerated the dead body, and this must have influenced their knowledge of pathologic anatomy. The value of this source of information was minimized, however, by the lowly status of this caste and the segregation of the priestly class, in whose hands the practice of medicine resided.* Lobstein quotes Pliny, on the other hand, to the effect that the Pharaohs attended autopsies: 'Iis (regibus) erat studium corpora scrutari mortuorum et causas valetudinis oculate fide recognoscere."† I have not been able to verify this quotation.

---

* See Dawson's "The Beginnings—Egyptian and Assyrian Medicine," Vol. I of this Series.
† Hist. Nat., Bk. IV, Ch. I (probably incorrect).

Our knowledge of Egyptian pathology comes largely from ancient papyri (Edwin Smith papyrus, 1600 B.C.; Ebers papyrus, 1550 B.C., and others). These are obviously based on much older writings of unknown date, so that the relative priority of Egyptian or Mesopotamian medicine cannot today be established. Interpretation of these old papyri is especially difficult because of our ignorance of the meaning of words obviously used by the Egyptians in a specific sense.

The Smith papyrus, though basically a clinical report on 48 surgical cases, shows that such pathological relationships as deafness following fracture of the temporal bone, a loss of speech from neck injuries, and paralysis from dislocation of the cervical vertebrae were recognized.

The Ebers papyrus, though devoting much space to illogical and complicated remedies, mentions many diseases, and details 47 actual cases—arthritis deformans, for instance, appearing as "hardening in the limbs"; other descriptions may reasonably be construed as indicating benign and malignant tumors, while diseases of the external organs, as might be expected, receive especial attention. Without too much stretch of the imagination, bilharzia and mastoid disease can be detected.

Judea. The pathological contributions of Jewish medicine were not inconsiderable. Rabbinical lore, acquired from shrewd observation of the sick and from food inspection, especially for reasons of public health, early produced much of value in the light of present-day knowledge. Details can be found in the interesting work of Preuss on Medicine in the Bible and the Talmud. It must be recognized, however, that the Jewish term for a given disease often included several clinical entities and that often the nature of the disease is largely conjectural. Thus "Zarasth," often translated as leprosy, probably included psoriasis, eczema, boils, maggoty sores or even syphilis.

Indian medicine, especially weak in its anatomy (because of the religious prohibition of dissection) and fanciful in physiology, was at first entirely theurgic. Later it regarded disease as an upset in the balance of moral and physical qualities (*nidana*). These latter consisted, at different times, of three (spirit, bile and phlegm) or seven fundamental properties (blood, flesh, fat, bone, bone marrow, chyle and semen). Though diseases were fantastically subdivided (Susruta, who flourished in the fifth century A.D., mentions 1120), nevertheless careful observation permitted advances well beyond the ordinary stages of folk medicine. Fever was regarded as "the king of all diseases"; the other chief diseases, according to Atreya tradition, as found in the Charaka Samhita, being the blood-bile disease (*rakta-pitta*), swelling (*gulma*), polyuria (*prameha*) (twenty kinds), leprosy (*kustha*), "darre," delirium (*unmada*) and unconsciousness (*apasmara*). Various infectious diseases were recognized, such as phthisis, smallpox and malaria (said to be attributed by Susruta to mosquitos). To Susruta is ascribed the earliest description of cholera; he emphasized the cyanosis, vomiting, prostration, emaciation and stupor. *Madhumeha,* "honey urine," and its chief symptoms suggest a knowledge of diabetes mellitus, though Reinhold Mueller points out that the sweetness was looked upon as occurring in the underlying substances. The surgical methods of Susruta show that, empirical and sacerdotal though the basis was, nevertheless a fairly adequate concept was held of the nature of suppuration, formation of calculi, granulation tissue, healing of fractures and other fundamental processes.

Early *Chinese*, and its offshoot early *Japanese*, medicine contain little of interest for the student of pathology. The lack of a firm anatomical basis, together with an extreme penchant for the influence of numbers and the usual rôle of superstition, produced purely fanciful theories of disease with especial over-elaboration of the pulse-lore and the indications for acupuncture. Disease was regarded as the lack of balance of the effects of the male and female principles, which were distributed to the various organs in methods corresponding to the government of the Celestial Kingdom. The various fevers alone were reckoned in the thousands.*

Greece. The golden age of Greece had its triumphs in medicine no less than in most fields of human endeavor; but they were not in the domain of pathologic anatomy. Hippocratic practice, however, was grounded so thoroughly on observation that fortunately its purely theoretical basis, the celebrated Humoral Doctrine, did little to help or harm.

Of unknown antiquity, this theory of the four humors: blood, phlegm, yellow and black bile, not only served the Greeks, the Romans and the medieval period, but its influence persisted, in

* See Morse's volume on "Chinese Medicine" in this Series.

part at least, practically till the establishment of
the cellular theory in the nineteenth century.
From the historical point of view, therefore, it
may be regarded as the most important of all
pathological concepts. According to Elgood*, this
doctrine "was taught in unmistakable terms in
the holy books of the Hindus" (prior to 2000
B.C.). From India it was carried to the Greeks by
way of Persia. Stated in simplest terms there were
four humors, just as there were four elements
of the philosophy of Empedocles: air, water, fire
and earth, and these humors consisted of mixtures of the four qualities: cold, heat, wetness
and dryness. Thus the blood, like air, was hot
and wet, the phlegm was cold and wet like water;
the yellow bile was hot and dry like fire; the
black bile (literally, "melancholy") was cold
and dry, like earth. The blood arose from the
heart, the phlegm ("*pituita*," hence pituitary
body) from the brain, the yellow bile from the
liver, the black bile from the spleen and the
four make up the nature of the body, φυσίς
(Hippocrates' Nature of Man, IV, 3). "San-
guine," "phlegmatic," "jaundiced," "melancholic," "venting one's spleen" are common
terms that are still used in the Greek humoral
sense. A proper balance and mingling of the
humors (εὐκρασία) maintained health
(ὑγίεια); an imbalance (δυσκρασία) (and especially a predominance of the black bile) produced disease. The idea of the mucus, or *pituita*,
flowing through the body, called by Hippocrates
"catarrh," persisted until 1660, when overthrown
by *Conrad Victor Schneider* (1614-80) of
Schneiderian membrane fame ("De catarrhis").

* See his "Medicine in Persia" in this Series.

The natural forces in the human body were regarded as tending to maintain εὐκρασία in spite of the opposing forces of disease. It is, by the way, an interesting study to consider the ingenuity with which newly observed phenomena were fitted through the centuries into this purely speculative theory. In it acute diseases were regarded as passing through three natural processes: (1) the prodromal or crude stage (apepsis); (2) that of ripening (coction, cooking of the humors—pepsis); (3) crisis or resolution, when as the result of a struggle the diseased material was expelled from the body by some natural avenue. "Diseases arise in some cases from regimen, in other cases by the air."* Hippocrates recognized that when an epidemic disease was prevalent it was due not to regimen but to some "unhealthy exhalation" in the air, though the opinion was also held among the Greeks that a widespread change of humoral balance had rendered the people susceptible.

Disease pictures that were recognizable by clinical observation were recorded by the Greeks in large and important numbers; those which could be elicited by post mortem study, on the other hand, are conspicuous by their absence; and this is not surprising as, except during the Alexandrian period, dissection was limited to animals and then for anatomical rather than pathological study. Thus from the Hippocratic period we get such clear pictures of healing of wounds by first and second intention, of the symptoms of suppuration, phthisis, gout, apoplexy, jaundice, cirrhosis of the liver, tetanus,

* Hippocrates' "Nature of Man," IX, 12.

diphtheria, quinsy, puerperal sepsis, mumps, various types of malaria, pneumonia, empyema, the "sacred disease" (epilepsy), various forms of tumors (see Chapter VII) and many other diseases that at least something of their general nature must have been fairly well recognized. It is hard for one who is not a Greek student to appreciate the many names of diseases that have remained unchanged for over 2000 years, until he compares the original with a translation of Hippocrates such as that of Jones in the Loeb classical library. On the other hand, such terms as the "coeliac passion" and the "iliac passion" were used by the Greeks, and for many centuries after, to cover in the one case most any condition causing a foul diarrhea; and, in the other, many disorders such as appendicitis, obstruction, spasm and the dry gripes of lead poisoning. Hippocrates had some conception at least of the antagonism of one disease for another, a problem still of interest and largely unsolved: he states, for instance, that patients with quartan fever do not get epilepsy; but, if they get epilepsy first and then quartan they will recover from the epilepsy —a strangely modern ring to this. Further, "Alcippo sickened with maniacal attacks, then an acute fever supervened and the attacks ceased"; yet the hyperthermic treatment of various psychoses is a product of the twentieth century.

Of the Alexandrian School, *Herophilus* and *Erasistratus* remain immortal, but more in anatomy and physiology than in pathology. Herophilus' four forces (nourishing, in the liver and digestive tract; warming, in the heart; mental, in the brain; and sensitive, in the nerves) had

little but a speculative basis and correspondingly
little future influence. His anatomical studies
he tried to correlate with disease (for instance,
he noted rupture of the ligamentum teres in dislocation of the hip) and he was said to be "the
first man who searched into the causes of disease"
by human dissections (Pliny), at some of which
Ptolemy was present. Though chiefly celebrated
as a physiologist, Erasistratus developed a theory
of disease based on "plethora" that is considered
in more detail in the next chapter. His oft-
quoted observation of accumulation of fluid in
the peritoneal cavity associated with hardness of
the liver (cirrhosis with ascites) is a splendid
early example of the value of the anatomical
study of disease.

The best account of Roman medicine, which
was so largely in the hands of or under the control of Greeks that it is impossible to separate
them, is from the pen of a non-medical patrician,
Cornelius Celsus (*ca.* 30 B.C.—*ca.* 38 A.D.). His
compilation, "De re medicina,"* ignored by his
medical contemporaries, is today an invaluable
record of the medical knowledge of the previous
centuries, and especially of the Alexandrian
School, whose original writings have been entirely lost. Beside his well-known signs of inflammation (see Chapter VII), he gave the
earliest description of rabies in man, mentions
a distemper of the large intestine on the right
side that is apparently appendicitis, considers
nasal polyp, nasal caries, enlarged tonsils, hernias, fatal otitis media, gonorrhea and soft
chancre and gives many other descriptions of
disease that have become classical.

* See recent translation in the Loeb series.

CHAPTER II

THEORIES OF THE NATURE OF DISEASE

THE various primitive theories of disease that might be included under the heading "demonic," and the classical Humoral Theory discussed in the last chapter are, from the point of view of the numbers of their supporters and years of dominance, the outstanding disease concepts throughout man's history. Numerous others, however, on account of their dominance over shorter periods of time and as interesting outcrops of the workings of ingenious medical minds, not only require description here but afford a valuable perspective for the present and future. The characteristic Greek tendency to theorize without sufficient observational basis led the followers of Hippocrates to split into many schools. The Dogmatists (Diocles, Praxagoras) especially emphasized theory, while the Empiricists based their treatment on previous experience without regard to logic or anatomic discoveries. *Erasistratus* (*ca.* 300 B.C.) of Cos, one of the chief glories of the Alexandrian School, though of course ignorant of the capillaries and the circulation of the blood, attributed practically all disease to a state of "plethora," which for him meant a stuffing of organs as well as vessels with an oversupply of nutritive material. It is easy to see how his observations on pneumonia and blood-spitting fitted such a scheme, while arthritis became due to a plethora of the joints, dropsy to a plethora of the liver, with other instances of the cart before the horse. Applications of this theory to inflammation and to ascites are discussed elsewhere; it had a surprising rebirth at the hands of Corvisart over two thousand years later.

Following the decline of Alexandria, the schools of Asia Minor dominated Greek medicine. Thence came *Asclepiades* of Bithynia (124 (?) -56 B.C.) who set up against the humoral doctrines of Hippocrates a *Solidism* which attributed disease to contracted or relaxed conditions of the solid parts: *strictum et laxum*, a view derived from the atomic theory of Democritus. This theory, which had various rebirths in the eighteenth-century views of Hoffmann, Brown and others, assumed a flow of vital fluids through an infinity of minute tubes or pores that connected the atoms that made up the body. If the normal relations were disturbed by constriction of the tubes, acute disease as a rule resulted; if by relaxation, the disease was usually chronic.

His pupils, *Themison* of Laodicea (123-43 B.C.) and others, enlarged the *strictum et laxum* theory to include increased or decreased excretion from the body. This *School of Methodism*, with its emphasis on atoms, held sway in Rome for over two centuries. Its consideration of the whole patient in relation to his environment connects it with the School of Cos, on the one hand, and with twentieth-century tendencies, on the other; but its disregard of local symptoms and the associated anatomical changes were sources of weakness that contributed to its decay.

The *Pneumatists,* led by *Athenaeus* of Attalia (*ca.* 70 B.C.) and *Archigenes* (*ca.* 54-117 A.D.), formed a third school of medical thought. For them the *pneuma,* or vital air, taken in by the lungs to cool the inner heat of the heart, was supreme. If disordered in quality or tone by a dyscrasia of the elements, disease resulted. Comparatively unimportant from an historical point of view, this school is supposed to have inspired much of the work of Aretaeus (second century) and Aetius (sixth century) and its doctrine appears again, in altered form, in the later views of Paracelsus and van Helmont.

Most of the prominent physicians of the early Christian era, *Rufus* (98-117), *Dioscorides* (first century), *Soranus* (second century), *Alexander of Tralles* (525-605), *Paul of Aegina* (502-575), were *Eclectics,* utilizing the best knowledge of their time, in somewhat the same sense as medical men of today accept proved advances without regard to their source.

In this period flourished *Galen* (*ca.* 130-200), the great Pergamene, who for his individual achievements as well as for the influence that he exerted over the civilized world's medicine for some 1500 years may well be regarded with Hippocrates as one of the two most important figures in all medical history. In fact the very strength of his teachings produced such an unquestioned dominance over centuries of medical thought that stagnation was bound to follow. This it is which is responsible for the widespread modern repugnance to "Galenism," meaning thereby a narrow dogmatism that was far from characteristic of its namesake. Galen's mistakes were numerous; but, in view of his limited opportunities, should be easily pardonable. His assertion of invisible pores in the ventricular septum, which proved such a stumbling block to the concept of the circulation of the blood; his belief in the need for suppuration ("coction") in the healing of wounds; and his adherence to the already ancient humoral doctrine of vital spirits, have blinded many to his extraordinary achievements in correlating the various branches of biology in their application to medicine, in experimental physiology, in comparative anatomy (especially of the pig and ape, human dissection being traditionally impossible) and in his diagnosis and treatment of disease.

Galen was philosophically an Eclectic who tried to avoid the errors of the various schools that preceded him. He appreciated the value of observation and experiment; but was sometimes led into error by his ardor to convert medicine into an exact science. His theory of disease, with which we are chiefly concerned here, was an extension of a numeralistic Humoralism combined with the dominance of the Pneuma. To the familiar four humors are added the three spirits: natural, πνεῦμα φύσικοη (from the liver to the body by the veins); vital, ζῶτικον (from the heart by the arteries); animal, ψύχικον (from the brain by the nerves), together with various subsidiary faculties and operations as detailed from Joannitius by Withington. Diseases were divided into three classes: (1) those affecting similar parts or simple tissues only (such as muscles, nerves); (2) organic (such as malformations and hypertrophies affecting compound tis-

sues) ; and (3) general (dyscrasias due to an imbalance of the humors, commonest among which
was an excess of black bile, the atrabilic group).
Causes of disease were predisposing (proegu-
menic), exciting (procatarctic), and coincident
(synectic). For health not only was the presentation (πρόσθεσις) of the several humors to the
various organs necessary in proper amounts, but
also their proper "adhesion" (πρόσσφυσις) was
essential; disease followed if either of these functions were deranged. Thus vomiting was interpreted as the result of failure of adhesion of food
to the digestive tract; edema as the failure of an
over-watery humor to adhere and be converted
into tissue juice; jaundice to the failure of the
spleen to remove the black bile (adhesion) normally present in the blood. Acute diseases usually
arose from disturbances of the blood and yellow
bile and characteristically stopped on the seventh
day; chronic diseases came from dyscrasias of
the phlegm and black bile.

Galen's views on the nature of disease are
scattered through his voluminous writings of almost 100 books; but his special pathology was
chiefly concentrated in the six books called "De
locis affectis." His concept of inflammations and
tumors (taken up in a later chapter) led him to
many deductions of practical value. Cholera,
hydrophobia and various forms of malaria were
well known to him; he knew of the relations of
urinary calculi to the kidney, ureter and bladder
and saw their resemblance to gouty deposits; he
recognized pus in the urine and often guessed
its site of origin; his views on nephritis were but

little improved on till the time of **Bright**; ozena, bronchitis, empyema, pleuritis, ulceration of the lung (with or without emaciation—phthisis) he accepted from the earlier Greeks, as he also did the explanation that "phymata" (tubercles) were due to coagulation of an over-viscid humor.*

Throughout the scientifically barren Dark and Middle Ages, Galenism was ever more unassailably enthroned in medical thought, so that even the occasionally observed fact was rejected if contrary to his written word. Contributions of the Arabs and of the many gifted Europeans during these centuries were only accepted if not in contradiction to Galen and his numerous commentaries, until the growing spirit of revolt from authority, characteristic of the Renaissance, produced such daring spirits as Paracelsus, who in 1527 formally burned the works of **Galen** and **Avicenna** in the Basel marketplace. Soon the anatomical concepts of disease, together with the more rational physiology initiated by **Harvey** and the students of respiration, were to offer a firm foundation for preferable theories; but there is danger of forgetting that Galenism continued to exert a predominant influence for more than a century after Harvey. In therapeutics it was the use of quinine in the early eighteenth century as a specific for malaria that struck the shattering blow—not annihilating, however, as our present methods of purging at the beginning of an illness and of increasing the elimination of toxic substances in acute diseases are of course strictly

* See also Lund's "Greek Medicine" in this Series and numerous articles by Joseph Walsh.

Galenical with but little improvement in verbiage or logical support.

While Arabian medicine is justly thought to be more famous in other fields than in pathology and is chiefly renowned as the preserver and transmitter of classical knowledge to the Renaissance, nevertheless the centuries of dominance of Avicenna's "Canon" would alone require that Arabian concepts of disease be recorded here. The Arabs accepted the Greek theory of the four humors (blood, phlegm, yellow and black bile) made of the four elements (earth, fire, air and water), each partaking of two of the four principles (hot, cold, dry, wet) ; also the three spirits: natural (seat in liver), vital (seat in heart), animal (seat in brain). While most diseases were thought to come from an imbalance or putrefaction of these humors, through obstruction to excretion of vapors, or by external influences such as excessive cold or moisture, they also considered the influence of infected air, parasites, poisons and improper nourishment. Gradually each organ, as well as each individual, came to be regarded as having its own constitution and perhaps its own tendency to disease (diathesis), which eventually became all important, so that in a given case the symptoms were fitted to the physician's ideas of the patient rather than to an established disease picture. According to Girardeau (Paris thesis, 1910), the cholemic diathesis was particularly stressed by the Arabs. Treatment, to be sure, was contingent on diagnosis—of the particular humor at fault; or of the organ at fault if the diagnosis was non-humoral. Accurate observations were not wanting,

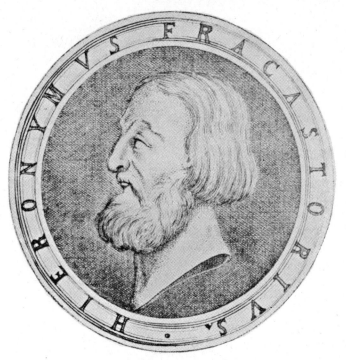

FIG. 2. Hieronymus Fracastorius.

such as those of Rhazes* on smallpox, measles, guinea-worm, spina ventosa; Haly Abbas on anthrax; Avicenna on diabetes, hemolytic versus obstructive jaundice; Albucasis on dental deformities; Avenzoar on the acarus of scabies, pericarditis, otitis media, mediastinal abscess. As against such real progress, of course, it must be recognized that astrology, irrational polypharmacy, uroscopy, religious convictions, charms, quackery and the like, all detracted enormously from the efficiency of medical practice, by the Europeans as well as the Arabs.

The encyclopedic knowledge and expository power of Avicenna's "Canon" made it the favorite textbook of medieval medicine, completely superseding the originals on which it was based. It was not until the ferment of the Renaissance condemned all medieval medical literature that the scholars of the time (Leonicenus, Linacre and a few others) set about substituting the originals of Hippocrates and Galen for the commentaries. Demonstration of the superiority of the Greek originals, not complete until the end of the sixteenth century, was perhaps a necessary prelude to the construction of the sound medical structure based on original observation and investigation that began with Vesalius and Harvey.

A brilliant light athwart the humoralism of the sixteenth century, before the anatomical idea had acquired much momentum, reaches us from the remarkable views on contagion of the Veronese, Hieronymus Fracastorius (ca. 1478†-1553),

---

* For Rhazes' experimental study of mercury poisoning in apes, see Elgood's "Persian Medicine." in this Series, p. 39.

† This is the date given by W. C. Wright (Hieronymi Fracastorii, N. Y., Putnam, 1930). The Encyclopedia Britannica gives 1483 and Garrison 1484 for Fracastorius' birth.

musician, poet, physicist, geologist and astronomer, as well as physician and pathologist. Far
more important than his better known poem,
"Syphilis sive morbus Gallicus" (1530), is his
later book, "De contagione et contagionis morbis
et curatione" (1546), which the Singers think
should earn for him the title of Father of Modern Pathology. Here, with remarkable insight,
he compares the virus of transmissible disease to
the fermentation of wine (*Cf.* Pasteur), and
writes of minute "seminaria contagionum,"
which, in spite of the obscurity of his description
and lack of microscopic support, have been interpreted as the first statement of the microbic origin of infectious disease. (See Athanasius
Kircher's "Scrutinium pestis" (1658) for the
first statement of *contagium animatum* supported by microscopic evidence.) In addition to
his scientific study of the eight contagious diseases
recognized in the Middle Ages (plague, phthisis,
epilepsy, scabies, erysipelas, anthrax, trachoma
and leprosy), he gave the first authentic account
of typhus fever, noting its contagiousness, re-
lating it to war and famine, and depicting
its peculiar rash. He described an epidemic of
hoof and mouth disease and wrote extensively on
syphilis (eventually accepting its venereal origin). He recognized three means of infection:
(1) by simple contact (as in scabies, phthisis and
leprosy); (2) by fomites (which carry the *"seminaria prima"*); and (3) by the air (smallpox,
plague, etc.) whence the "seminaria" are inhaled
and carried through the body by the humors for
which they have affinity.

The first openly to oppose Galen was the Swiss,

Aurelius Theophrastus Bombastus von Hohen-heim, better known as *Paracelsus** (1493-1541), whose works have recently been so thoroughly edited by Sudhoff. Whatever may have been the contributions of this great, practical but boastful, mystic in shaking the dominance of Galenism and in furthering the use of chemicals in therapy, his theories of diseases helped none but himself. Thus we read: "the Archaeus, or vital principle, the very essence of life, is enclosed in an invisible Mumia. In disease, the patient's Mumia must be transferred into the plant that bears the signature of that disease, in order to attract the specific influence from the stars, which govern all diseases." Yet only one of his five "entia" is astral, the *ens astrorum*; the other four being the *ens venenum* (the various internal and external poisons); *ens naturale* (diathesis from organic defects); *ens spirituale* (psychic); and *ens deale* (of divine origin). When through any or several of these causes an imbalance of normal functions occurred, disease was the result. As a practitioner, Paracelsus seems to have been active and efficient, and *inter alia* described fibroid phthisis in miners, linked cretinism with endemic goiter, recognized the precipitative nature of calculi and gouty deposits, and related paralysis and speech disturbances to injuries of the head. But above all to be credited to him was his important in-

---

* He seems to have a penchant for the prefix "Para," which he attached to subtitles of several of his works to form meanings that are still quite obscure. In the case of his name, it is thought by some to indicate "surpassing Celsus." "Aurelius" is said to have been added on account of his light yellow hair. The rest of the name he is entitled to by birth—our common noun, "bombast," being easy to derive from his temperamental display.

fluence on his contemporaries in revolting against blind authority and thus preparing the way for concrete scientific advances through independent observation.

An archaeus, this time named "Blas," also served the Belgian mystic, *van Helmont* (1577-1644), the founder of the Iatro-Chemical School, that sought to explain all things medical as chemical in nature. For van Helmont every bodily process was controlled by a Blas, these chemical processes being brought about each by a special ferment or "gas." (This is the first use of the term "gas" in science; it was derived from the old Greek word, *chaos*, as used by Paracelsus in the general sense of air.) When the vital body force in man, *archaeus insitus*, together with the *archaeus influus*, the divine force which regulates both physical and psychical activity, are upset by the *idea morbosa*, disease results. It is difficult to evaluate his mystical jargon, but he apparently conceived of disease as an actual but invisible principle ("Morbi prodeunt ab entibus conceptis, non a calore vel humore") endowed with diverse properties, and not as a state resulting from an imbalance of humors. Though his theories did little more than continue the Paracelsian revolt against Galen, he seems to have had considerable knowledge of secretory phenomena and an appreciation of the nature of infection and resistance to disease.

A more important supporter of the Iatro-Chemical School was the Hanoverian, *Franciscus Sylvius* (de la Boe) (1614-72), to whose lectures at Leiden students flocked from all Europe. Through his followers Willis, de Graaf, Stensen,

Swammerdam, Sennert and Boerhaave, his chemical theories of body function and his recognition of the importance of the blood in health and disease exerted widespread influence. He is credited with a knowledge of acidosis and alkalosis, thinking that acids and alkalis were balanced in the healthy body, but this was indeed a far cry from our understanding of these terms today. "If all the blood is black, that shows that acid predominates; if on the other hand it is red, bile predominates." Balance was restored by increasing excretion, but bloodletting was condemned.

Beside the anatomical discoveries which bear his name (the Fissure and the Aqueduct), and his chemical contributions, he performed many autopsies and especially advanced the subject of tuberculosis. He identified tubercles as related to phthisis (denied since the time of Aretaeus), recognized tuberculosis of lymph nodes and worked out the pathogenesis of cavities: "I found more than once larger and smaller tubercles in the lung, which on section were shown to contain pus. I believe that these tubercles become purulent and are changed into cavities, which are lined with this membrane. From these tubercles I hold that not infrequently phthisis has its origin." As Long says, "it is possible to construct a good working pathologic anatomy of tuberculosis from Sylvius' observations," which. were to be but little improved upon until the appearance of Laennec's immortal work.

Cornelius Bontekoe (1647-87), who wrote on "Die Lehre vom Alcali und Acido durch Wirckung der Fermentation und Effervescentz," asserted that thickening of the blood was the cause of all disease. Tea drinking, by thinning the blood, was therefore a panacea; but there is suspicion that he was in the pay of the newly prominent Dutch tea-merchants!

Thomas Willis (1621-75), the most prominent English Iatro-Chemist, as well as being a great clinician and contributor to normal anatomy (the Nerve and Circle of Willis), is important to pathology for his work on the nervous system ("Pathologiae cerebri et nervosi generis specimen," 1667), for his observation of sweetish urine in diabetes, his probable recognition of meningitis as a cause of convulsions, and his description of typhoid fever in the army ("epidemical dysentery"). He described scurvy, myasthenia gravis, and paresis and was the first to describe and name puerperal fever (Garrison). Living through troublous times, as a Royalist he was made Professor of Natural History at Oxford after the Restoration and continued his good work after moving to London in 1666, where he acquired a huge practice. How much of his achievement is owed to his assistant, Lower, is still a matter of lively discussion.

Opposed to the Iatro-Chemists was the Iatro-Physical (or Iatro-Mathematical) School, that sought to explain vital phenomena on the basis of physics. Beginning worthily with attempts at clinical thermometers, pulse clocks, and balances (who does not recall Sanctorius' famous metabolic studies on the "steelyard chair"?), they made the inestimable gift of quantitation to medical science. Harvey's great discovery was a shining example of what was to be accomplished in such ways. The master minds of Descartes and Borelli, the most prominent members of the school, contributed greatly to the physiology of the various systems of the body; but pathology profited less.

Giorgio Baglivi (1668-1706), the pupil of Malpighi who left us a description of the cerebral hemorrhage that caused his master's death, was the leading Italian representative of the school. Though he was an acute observer at the bedside and autopsy table, as a theorist he could do no better than to liken the human body to a group of machines: the teeth being the scissors, the stomach the flask, the chest a bellows, the heart and vessels the pump and pipes of a waterworks (Neuburger).

Thomas Sydenham (1624-89), a Roundhead captain of horse who acquired his doctorate at the age of fifty-two, though rightly ranked primarily as a practitioner of physic—the English Hippocrates, indeed—must also be given place in this description of theories of disease. Achieving the most important of the several returns to Hippocrates that are found in the history of medicine, he emphasized the value of observation and placed clinical experience above theory and the "preclinical branches." He was probably too much concerned with practical details always to maintain symmetry of theory; but some theory at least had to be subscribed to, even by Sydenham. As a humoralist, he conceived of disease as nature's effort to throw off the *materies morbi*, even though his therapeutics included the use of cinchona, iron, mercury, laudanum, adjuvant purges and general hygienic measures. Each disease was thought of as an independent natural process, coming from outside the body and following a natural course, though diseases could be grouped like plants and were subject to change by seasonal and atmospheric influences ("epidemic constitutions"). The actual development of acute diseases he believed to be due to inflammation of the blood for reasons that he thought too obscure to be worth investigation; chronic diseases were due to humors disordered by diet or habits of life and therefore our own fault: *"Acutos dico, qui ut plurimum Deum habent authorem, sicut chronici ipsos nos."* Concretely, he first separated scarlatina (which he named) from measles (1675), first described the form of chorea that bears his name (1686) and wrote masterly descriptions of gout (1683), hysteria, smallpox and other diseases. A sesquicentennial recrudescence of his influence will be found in the English and Irish schools of the early nineteenth century.

Of a somewhat similar type and of far greater influence on European medicine was *Hermann Boerhaave* (1668-1738), the Batavian Hippocrates, *communis totius Europae praeceptor* (Haller). A letter from a Chinese mandarin "To the illustrious Boerhaave, physician in Europe," is said to have reached him without delay. A believer, like Hippocrates, in the prime importance of clinical observation, in theory an eclectic, he made selections both from the Iatro-Physicists and Iatro-Chemists. He took into consideration diseases of the solid parts as well as of the humors. Disorders of the humors were both quantitative and qualitative in nature; in the solid tissues, significant were changes in form, in size, in consistency and in content of the blood vessels—before Morgagni, a clinician could hardly be expected to go much further. He recognized the value of postmortem examinations and published at least two important accounts of autopsies from his own practice (rupture of the esophagus, cardiac dilatation and suffocation from a fatty tumor of the mediastinum). Expanding the method of bedside instruction which he received from Montanus through his predecessors, Schrevelius and Heurnius, he made Leyden the center of medical instruction in Europe. Through his Edinburgh disciples, he directly influenced the development of medicine in America, as Welch has pointed out, as well as fathering through van Swieten and deHaen the hegemony of the "Old Vienna School."

In the eighteenth century, the age of systems, more than one speculative theory of diseases achieved undeserved prominence. One such was the "animistic" theory of *George Ernest Stahl* (1660-1734), which with the "tonus" theory of his erstwhile friend Friedrich Hoffmann dominated most of eighteenth century medicine. Stahl, in opposition to Descartes' mechanistic views, and somewhat in the sense of Aristotle's *psyche* or van Helmont's *archaeus*, conceived of the *anima* as the life force (an idea nearer to the sum total of natural forces than to our ideas of mind or soul) which governed the activities of the living body and protected it against the tendency to degenerate. It normally produced in the body a series of movements which constituted health. When these were disorganized disease resulted, which was looked upon as the tendency to restore orderly motion. This took place chiefly through the circulatory system, so that especial attention was paid to the increased pulse rate of febrile diseases. When the *anima* left the body or any of its parts, putrefaction resulted. Acting on the humoral concept that disease developed in the blood, Stahl believed plethora (due to atony) to be of great importance, and he therefore let blood freely. He committed the error of denying the value of opium and cinchona. He was also responsible for introducing the term "phlogiston" into science in 1702, in his edition of Becher. This much debated concept was expanded in his "Opuscula chymica physico-medico," 1715. A great teacher and a prolific writer, with over 300 publications to his credit, Stahl exerted an enormous influence on his contemporaries, an influence that is traced by Garrison to Whytt, Bichat and even the "Entelechies" of Dreisch, while Castiglioni regards him as the first to have given a biologic trend to medicine.

Friedrich Hoffmann (1660-1742), a colleague of Stahl on the Halle faculty and born in the same year, the friend of Boyle and Ramazzini, was another to develop an influential theory of disease, one similar to the *strictum et laxum* of Asclepiades: Force being inherent in matter, life consists of motion; cessation of motion is death. The body was looked upon as made up of fibers which have characteristic tonuses, which make them contract and dilate. The tonus is maintained and regulated by a nervous ether, which is sent forth from the brain by pulsating messages throughout the body. Disease is caused by changes of tonus, chiefly due to plethora. Acute disease is due to spasm; chronic disease to atony. But disordered humors and excretions also contribute, hence in treatment sedatives, "tonics" (a relic that persists in our vocabulary today), alteratives and Galenical evacuants were employed. Hoffmann's anodyne is still in use. Also a prolific writer, Hoffmann is regarded by Garrison as "a great, original physician, whose writings await intensive study," and by Allbutt as the greatest of the Iatro-Physicists, the first to perceive that "pathology is an aspect of physiology."

Jerome David Gaub (Gaubius) (1705-80), Boerhaave's successor at Leyden, is an interesting example of how the most successful teacher of pathology of his day in Europe continued the sterile exposition of a modified humoral theory, blind to the growing accumulation of pathologico-anatomical knowledge that is to be described in the next chapter. His widely read book, "Institutiones pathologiae medicinalis," (1758) a systematic treatise designed apparently for his student auditors, first appeared three years before Morgagni's "De sedibus," but was continued unchanged in several editions for another score of years. We search through it in vain for the solid facts that had accumulated in the previous century. Pathology, the theory of the morbid states of man, to be sure, is stated as treating of disordered function as well as structure, the divisions of general and special pathology are considered and its causes are subdivided into the familiar predisposing and active, remote and proximal (we even read of hormones and animate causes of disease), but no meat clings to these dry bones. "Chemical analysis" of the body shows that it is composed of wet substance (the most mobile), inflammable (the food of fire), saline (the friend of water) and earthy (resisting fire and water). Disease comes from improper mixtures of these: putridity, for instance, is a kind of corruption that easily ensues if there is a copious supply of wet and inflammable. Deficiency of the natural cohesion of the body matter causes debility, tenuity or dissolution (hemorrhages, diarrhea, ptyalism, pustules); excessive cohesion causes undue tenacity, "spissitude" (stagnation, obstruction, infarction, tumors). We hopefully meet "aneurysma," "anastomosis," only to find that they are diseases of the contents of solid structures, or cavities which admit or emit too much laxity! In the discussion of coagulation of the blood (in which its microscopic appearance is mentioned) we learn that increase of its watery constituent gives the phlegmatic temperament; of its fibrous density, the melancholic; and of its red portion (phlogiston), the choleric. Among the animate causes of disease that pervade air, earth and water, are "very minute animalculae" in stupendous numbers which multiply so quickly that they have multifarious occasions when they can harm man. At this interesting point, however, the lecturer passes on to intestinal worms, whose origin he suspects may be from natural putridity, from "the arbitrary spirit of the world," from some seed introduced into the body or some change in the food. And so on through 512 pages that were deservedly discarded soon after the author's death. They would not merit the space given them here, if it were not to emphasize the archaic nature of pathologic teaching at a time when Morgagni was ready to publish his encyclopedic observations on gross pathology and Auenbrugger his discovery of percussion, when Haller had largely completed his physiological masterpieces and John Hunter was actively engaged in the development of experimental biology.

Of different caliber was the vulgar *John Brown* (1735-88), whose Brunonism dominated large groups of medical thought into the nineteenth century. Though announced in 1780 in his "Elementa medicinae" (1780), nineteen years after Morgagni's "De sedibus," his theory applied Haller's views on irritability to the thesis that health consisted in a constant succession of balanced stimuli from the exterior, which, if excessive, produces sthenic diseases; if insufficient, asthenic diseases. Opium and alcohol were the panaceas. Brunonism is chiefly important to us for the enthusiasm with which it was accepted abroad: by Benjamin Rush in this country, by Rasori (who translated the "Elementa") and others in Italy, by Broussais in France, and by numerous others in Austria and Germany. Broussais regarded heat as the all-important vital factor, through its stimulation of the chemical processes of the body. Disease was due to the local irritation of an organ, but especially of the gastrointestinal tract. Gastroenteritis, therefore, was the all-important disease, to be fought by a slender, antiphlogistic diet, and by withdrawal of bad blood by leeches. Baas states that "in the

year 1833 alone 41½ million leeches were im-
ported into France!" This welter of blood, increased by Broussais' pupil, Bouillaud, continued until overthrown by Louis in 1835 on the
basis of careful statistics ("Récherches sur les
effets de la saignée"). The contribution that the
statistical method, which was thus inaugurated,
still continues to make to the medical sciences
would require a book of its own for adequate
evaluation.

One more "system" was to exert considerable
influence. Strangely enough it was proposed after
the Cell Theory had been announced and
not long before the dawn of Cellular Pathology,
by one of the greatest of all pathologists—Carl
Rokitansky: the theory of crases—plastic lymph—
and dyskrases, which will be taken up in a later
chapter.

But the day of dominance of speculative theories was drawing to a close. Henceforth they
might occasionally have their vogue, but the
ever-swelling volume of a rationally based system was becoming too great to be materially ob-
structed. In fact the effect of these new systems,
though founded on illogical or even absurd be-
liefs, has often been to correct the very errors in
the medical practice of the time that allowed
them to take root. Thus, with Mesmerism, *Franz
Mesmer* (1734-1815) called attention to the aid
that may be got from hypnotism and suggestion,
and the absurdly minute doses of the Homeop-
athy of *Christian Frederick Samuel Hahnemann*
(1755-1843) went far to correct the current evils
of polypharmacy of that day. In our own day

Osteopathy will doubtless lead to a better appreciation of the value of proper manipulation and massage, just as Christian Science has shown the importance of the patient's mental attitude in combating a wide variety of physical disorders.

CHAPTER III

THE RISE OF ANATOMIC CONCEPTS IN DISEASE

DURING the 1500 years or more that the theoretical explanations of the causes of diseases held sterile sway, it was inevitable that valuable isolated pathologic observations should have been made, some of which have already been referred to. Indeed, as we have seen in the previous chapter, old false theories maintained their ground or new ones continued to be promulgated long after a sound basis of pathologic anatomical study had been laid. Nevertheless, a fairly distinct period can be marked out where the importance of the tissue changes produced by disease (i.e., lesions) began to be recognized and the attempt made to explain both the nature of the disease and its symptoms by study of these lesions.

Postmortem examinations seem to have been made through the centuries (often in cases of suspected poisoning), though it is hard at this distance always to distinguish "anatomies," or dissections, from the examinations made to ascertain the cause of death. Morgagni speaks of necropsies performed in Byzantium in the sixth century to investigate the cause of plague, and Chiari—at about third hand, to be sure—tells of a physician of Cremona who performed many autopsies in the plague of 1286. We know that *William of Saliceto* (*ca.* 1201-80) performed at least one medicolegal necrospy, that on the nephew of the Marchese Pallavicini; and, as Long points out, the first book of Saliceto's "Summa conservationis" (1275) is practically a book of special pathology, containing *inter alia* a reference to sclerotic kidneys ("durities in renibus") and correlating kidney disease with the onset of dropsy. *Bartolomeo da Varignana,* pupil of the celebrated Bolognese anatomist, Taddeo Alderotti, investigated in 1302, at the court's order, the suspicious death of a nobleman named Azzolino, the report of which autopsy is still extant. Doubtless such procedures were not infrequent. Even the most exalted were examined: In 1410 Pope Alexander v dying suddenly and therefore under suspicious circumstances, his body was "posted" by *Pietro d'Argelata,* a surgeon who was Guy de Chauliac's most distinguished pupil.

Mundinus (Mondino de'Luzzi) (*ca.* 1275-1326?) , another pupil of Taddeo's, wrote in 1316 a small "Anathomia," that to be sure included the errors of Galen and the Arabists on which it was based, but nevertheless was destined to exert for over two centuries a great influence on anatomic development. He and his pupil Bertuccio (the teacher of Guy de Chauliac) included a number of pathologic observations in their works (Chiari) . Public dissections were soon after authorized in all the leading medical centers; the anatomic theater of Padua was built in 1490, and necropsies are known to have been authorized or performed in Venice, Florence, Siena and Montpellier in the fourteenth century and in Vienna, Bologna, Padua, Prague, Paris and Tübingen in the fifteenth century (Garrison) .

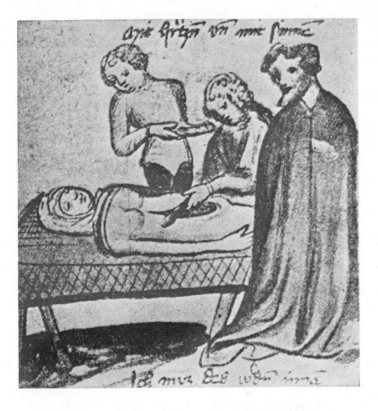

FIG. 3. A Fourteenth Century German Autopsy.
(From the "Welt Chronik" of Rudolf of Ems.)

Nevertheless, these advances seemingly accomplished little more than to prolong the errors of Galen and Mundinus and it was not until the basis of a correct human anatomy had been laid that sound observations in pathologic anatomy could be expected.

The publication, then, of Vesalius' "De fabrica humani corporis" (1543) constitutes not only one of the shining achievements of the Renaissance of learning but also the most important medical event in the 1300 years since the work of Galen.*

But few pre-Vesalian figures need detain us in our pathologic survey. Of prime importance, however, is *Antonio Benivieni (ca.* 1440-1502), an able Florentine surgeon, who described some twenty postmortem incisions made specifically to determine the cause of death and explain symptoms. These, included in 111 short chapters, were published posthumously (1507) under the title "De abditis causis morborum." Emphasis has rightly been placed on the effort to explain the hidden or internal causes of disease. Hecker called Benivieni the father of pathologic anatomy and Garrison regarded him as "the founder of pathology before Morgagni." Allbutt is even more enthusiastic: "Before Vesalius, before Eustachius, he opened the bodies of the dead as deliberately and clearsightedly as any pathologist in the spacious times of Baillie, Bright and Addison." Malgaigne's appreciation of his book "as the only book on pathology that owes nothing to anyone," is less open to dispute. The book begins conventionally with a discussion of the

* See Corner's "History of Anatomy," in this Series.

morbus Gallicus, but goes on to give short descriptions of what are obviously cases of pyloric carcinoma, acute pericarditis, cholelithiasis, abscess of the hip joint, "that black ulcer which the Greeks call gangrene," various hernias and fistulas, and so on. As the book is excessively rare, Long has performed a welcome service in translating some of the more interesting cases for his "Selected Readings in Pathology."

Following close on Benivieni was another Italian, *Alessandro Benedetti* (*ca.* 1460-1525), who built the celebrated anatomic theater at Padua, which included among its illustrious names those of Vesalius, Columbus, Fabricius of Aquapendente, Harvey and Morgagni. Author of an "Anathomia" in 1497, Benedetti also recorded various pathologic observations (gallstones, apoplexy, malposition of heart) and gave an important stimulus to the anatomical point of view in disease.

Surgeons have always had more or less opportunity to see pathologic lesions in the living state. Thus *Guy de Chauliac* (*ca.* 1300-68), the most erudite surgeon of his time, distinguished the various kinds of hernia from varicocele, hydrocele and sarcocele. *Bartolomeo Montagna* (died *ca.* 1460), who performed fourteen dissections, described various heart lesions, also ureteral stricture, while *Antonio Guanerio* (died 1440), *Michele Savonarola* (died 1462) (grandfather of the heretic) and *Giovanni Arcolani* (died *ca.* 1480) are said by Chiari to have reported pathologic observations. *Berengario da Carpi* (1470-1550), professor of Surgery at Bologna, is said to have made over 100 dissections, though some of these, like Galen's, may have been on pigs. His illustrated commentary on Mundinus (1521), one of the great pre-Vesalian texts, includes pathologic observations, as well as the more important anatomical observations on the valves of the heart, the vermiform appendix, the ventricles of the brain and the pineal gland.

While postmortem dissection was rare, human vivisection was apparently not unknown. Vesalius, Fallopius and Berengarius were all accused of this practice, but probably with injustice. As is apparent from the explanations of Berengarius, his "anatomia in vivis," the "living pathology" of today's surgical operation, was later taken to mean vivisection. Nevertheless, Fioravanti stated that he had seen living men dissected at Rome and that he himself had dissected the living in the wars against the Moors.*

While the sixteenth century saw the foundation of a true anatomy, with such giants as Vesalius, Realdus Columbus, Canano, Fallopius, Eustachius and Fabricius of Aquapendente coming readily to mind, it must also be remembered that those were the days of universalism. The same men were often the chief contributors to several branches of the healing art, such as medicine, surgery, obstetrics and, not the least among the various branches, to pathologic anatomy.

Within eleven years of the publication of the "Fabrica" appeared the first great work to profit by the new order. *Jean Fernel* (1497-1558), mathematician, astronomer, philosopher, physician to Henry II, and to Henry's wife and mis-

* See Giordano, I Cong. de l'Hist. de l'Art de Guérir, Lib. Mem., 1920, p. 65.

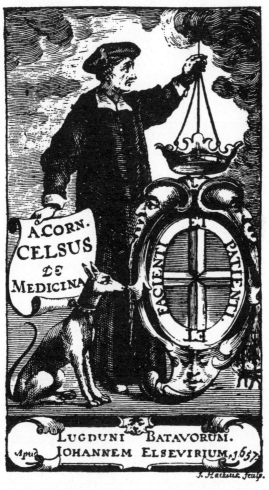

FIG. 4. Jean Fernel, as he appears on the title page of the
Elzevir edition of Celsus' "De re medicina."

tress as well, one of the great minds of a great century, in 1554 published his "Universa medicina." This great work, divided into three parts: physiology, pathology and therapeutics, was, as has been well brought out by Long, of prime importance to European medicine in developing a rational pathological viewpoint. A practitioner rather than a professional anatomist, Fernel nevertheless exhibits to us a rich store of morbid anatomical facts in his "Pathologiae libri vii," "the first medical work to be called a text of Pathology" (Long). Among many other valuable items are the first description of appendicitis ("iliac passion"), "obstruction (by sand, calculus and viscid humor), scirrhous inflammation, abscess and ulcer" of liver and kidneys, emphasis on the reciprocal relation of urine and sweat and the importance of an abnormal quantity of urine, ureteral dilatation, "abscess" of the stomach (which included both ulcer and cancer), various uterine disorders, "sarcoma" (i.e., any chronic superficial nodular mass such as chronic granulation tissue, polyps, true skin sarcomata, etc.), "vomica" of the lungs (probably including true abscess, gangrene and tuberculous cavities) and syphilis in various manifestations. In his nosology a Galenist, and often spoken of as the French Galen, in spite of his appreciation of the changes in the tissues, Fernel subscribed to the theory of the four humors, coction and the rest, and to most of what the theory implied. Yet his systematic handling of disease constituted perhaps his most useful contribution. General diseases were those of general distribution and uncertain sites ("morbi incertae sedis"), such as

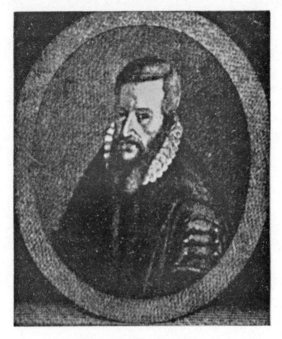

FIG. 5. Volcher Coiter.

the fevers (simple, putrid and pestilential). The special diseases (of known location) were classified as: (1) those above the diaphragm; (2) below the diaphragm; (3) external; and subdivided into: (1) simple (involving part of an organ); (2) compound (involving a whole organ); and (3) complicated (involving more than one organ). In each class, the organs were taken up *seriatim*, a method followed with but few exceptions from the Smith papyrus up to the latest textbooks of pathology.

The professional anatomists were also steadily advancing the anatomical concept of disease, since they, like the biochemists of today, were almost as much concerned with the abnormal as the normal. This concept was chiefly promoted in the sixteenth century by a Swiss, a Dutchman and an Italian, *Felix Plater, Volcher Coiter* and *Marcello Donato*. All of these, like the well-known Swiss, *Bauhinus,* the Dutchman, *Pieter Paauw* and the Spaniard, *Valverde,* had been students in Italy and through Fallopius and others may be regarded as direct inheritors of the Vesalian tradition. *Plater* (1536-1614), who, according to Chiari, dissected more than 300 bodies in fifty years, made numerous pathologic observations (e.g., "stone beneath the tongue," giantism, enlarged thymus, intestinal parasites, cystic liver and kidney). His two chief works "De partium corporis humani structura et usu libri III," and "Observationes in hominis affectibus" etc. exerted great influence for two centuries. *Volcher Coiter* of Groningen (1534-90), who taught at Bologna and practiced in Nuremberg, was especially noted for his work on ankylosis,

on the osteology of children and animals and
on exudates of the brain and spinal cord (meningitis) . His experiments on decapitated animals
are still remembered. He was a thorough believer
in the importance of pathologic anatomy and
was successfully insistent with the civil authorities on the need for autopsies in the study of disease. So, too, was the Italian, *Marcello Donato,*
(fl. end of sixteenth century) whose views on the
subject are quoted by Renouard and Long. For
the similar and only slightly less important contributions of *Giulio Cesare Aranzi* (1530-89) ,
Franciscus Vallesius (?-1592) , *Amatus Lusitanus*
(1511-?) , *Rembert Dodoens* (1517-85) , *Pieter
van Foreest* (1522-97) and others, we must refer
to larger works. One other, *Johann Schenck von
Grafenberg* (1530-98) must, however, receive a
few words, if only for his happy faculty of pre-
serving for us the many pathologic observations
that would otherwise be buried deep in anatomical and medical texts of previous writers. In
Book 2 of his observations, he quotes a hundred
or more authorities, one-half of them "recent"—
much the same group as one would select today
for the period covered. A practicing physician of
Strassburg and Freiburg, in 1597 he published
his "Observationum medicorum rararum . . .
libri vii," which combined his own extensive experiences with many concise pathologic reports
from practically all the important works since
classical times, all classified and indexed in an
orderly manner. Among others, may be cited his
reference to Avenzoar's "verruca ventriculi,"
Bauhinus' finding of cerebral hemorrhage and
Garnerus' case of splenomegaly (probably mye-

loid leucemia) (Long). Schenck also supports
his views on the value of postmortem examinations by numerous quotations.

As in the fourteenth and fifteenth centuries,
so in the sixteenth did surgeons with their access
to the "living pathology" continue to contribute
notably to morbid anatomy. In Italy, *Giovanni
Filippo Ingrassia* (1510-80) made some of the
earliest studies of bone lesions and of the effect
of synostoses and is also said to have been the
first to describe varicella (1553). In France, the
great and picturesque surgeon, *Ambroise Paré*
(1510-90), advanced knowledge of the nature of
disease by his insistence on the healing powers of
Nature ("Je le pansay, Dieu le guarit") ; he also
disproved the current idea that gunshot wounds
were poisonous by forbidding their preliminary
treatment with boiling oil. His treatise on monsters (1573) (imaginary as well as authentic)
and his description of monoxide poisoning
(1575) are of more strictly pathological concern,
while his popularization of Vesalius' "Fabrica"
by the publication of an epitome in the vernac-
ular was influential for the progress of anatomical concepts. As the first to see flies as trans-
mitters of disease (H. Kelly), he was far ahead
of his times. In Germany, *Fabricius Hildanus*
(1560-1634) emphasized the importance of normal and morbid anatomy. Though a believer in
setons, cautery and weapon salves (applied to the
weapon not the wound!), he wrote well on burns
(separating the still current three degrees) and
on gangrene. In his century of surgical cases he
discussed pathologic anatomy and physiology as
well as diagnosis and treatment. In England,

Richard Wiseman (1622-76) was soon to contribute to pathology with his descriptions of *"tumor albus"* (tuberculosis of the joints), the "King's Evil" and gonorrheal stricture, which he treated by external urethrotomy.

Marco Aurelio Severino (1580-1656), surgeon and professor of anatomy at Naples, not only wrote notably (if often incorrectly) on neoplasms and syphilis, but in his famous "De recondita abscessuum natura" (1632) was the first to include illustrations of lesions with his text. This book, which Long regards as the first text of Surgical Pathology, treats of all sorts of swellings under the term "abscess," so that it is not to be wondered at that their nature seemed recondite 300 years ago! Among neoplasms, Severinus describes those of the genital organs of both sexes and sarcomata of bones; and in his classification of four types of breast tumors differentiates between benign and malignant types. These four types, however: glandular, strumous, scirrhous and cancerous, are obscure terms and certainly have different meanings from those they have today. Another of his works, "Zootomia democritae" (1645), was one of the earliest descriptions of pathologic anatomy.

In Amsterdam, *Nicolas Tulp* (1593-1674), a pupil of Pieter Paauw and the central figure of Rembrandt's celebrated painting, The Lesson in Anatomy, contributed to pathology in his "Observationes medicae" (Elzevier, 1641 and 1672). He gave clear descriptions of carcinomas of the bladder and esophagus, of hydatidiform mole, and beriberi (ten years after Bontius). The illustrations in the book show a nasal polyp, a fibrinous bronchial cast (which he took to be vessels) , an expectorated fragment of gangrenous lung, various tapeworms (depicted with ferocious heads!) and calculae and monsters, a good spina bifida, a chimpanzee (which he first described) and a swordfish. Like Bauhinus, and many others before and after, he described and pictured an intracardiac clot as a "polypus cordis" without suspecting its postmortem origin.

Another to apply successfully the newly won anatomy to pathologic problems was the Dane, *Thomas Bartholin* (1616-80) . Son of a distinguished scholar, Caspar, he was a good representative of the peripatetic universalist; Leyden, Paris, Montpellier, Padua, Basel, all found him studying and teaching such diverse subjects as philosophy (which, to be sure, included much of the biology of the day) , ethics, theology, mathematics and medicine. His "Historiarum anatomicarum et medicarum rariorum centuriae v et vi," and his "Epistolae" contain many pathologic observations, both from clinical and postmortem cases, but so uncritically thrown together with superstitions and impossibilities that they lose much of their value. We find good descriptions of aortic arteriosclerosis, urinary calculi, anomalies of the nails, brain abscess following fracture of the skull, polyuria with disease of the pancreas, transudates in pleural, pericardial and peritoneal cavities in heart disease, but with no attempt to correlate cause and effect. His projected "Anatomia practica," a systematic collection of pathologic findings in all organs, was frustrated by the destruction of his papers when his house burned down.

Apoplexy, with its striking signs, had concerned the ancients since the time when Nabal became as a stone for ten days before he died (I Samuel, xxv, 37). Hippocrates, Lucretius, Galen, Celsus, Paul of Aegina and others had observed its phenomena and estimated the prognosis; but the condition was confused with syncope, with other paralyses, aphonias and sudden deaths and the explanation of the cause had been quite fanciful (obstruction of the pneumatic humor in its passage from the ventricles, for instance), until put on a firm basis by the clinico-pathologists of the seventeenth century. Chief among these was *Johann Jakob Wepfer* (1620-95) whose postmortem studies clearly revealed the causative relation of hemorrhage beneath the dura and into the ventricles and substance of the brain. In his "Observationes anatomicae ex cadaveribus eorum quos sustulit apoplexia" (Schaffhausen, 1658) 4 such cases with clinical and autopsy findings are admirably reported. Other lesions, such as rupture of an abscess into the ventricles, had already been noted to cause similar pictures; thus Plater (Observationes, Lib. I, p. 13) speaks of a "tumor" in the cerebrum, Bartholin (Cent. 4, Observ. 86) of apoplexy, fatal in three days, resulting from removal of a tumor, Willis (De anima brutorum, p. 21) of a meningeal abscess rupturing into the brain, and Ballonius (Definit. Med., p. 94) of an ear abscess rupturing internally. But it is apparent that these were not apoplexy in the modern sense. Wepfer's discovery was not one of chance.

He was a famous physician who recognized the great value of necropsies and went to great trouble in procuring them; and his achievement stands out as a bright beacon on the tortuous pathway of pre-Morgagnian pathology. When he died from "asthma," his own body was examined "as customary" (!) , and extensive sclerosis and calcifications of the aorta were found.

Thus by the seventeenth century the anatomical concept of disease and the study of its effects on the solid parts may be considered as well under way. Still consisting of sporadic and unsystematic observations, it laid the necessary foundations for the organized adequate consideration of gross morbid anatomy, to be described in the next chapter. Benefiting from the new anatomical knowledge initiated by Vesalius' "Fabrica" and indirectly and to a lesser extent from Harvey's demonstration of the circulation of the blood, it nevertheless still operated for the most part under the handicap of Galenic concepts of the causes and nature of disease. It is not surprising that, with such inadequate concepts of disease, fundamental advances in the treatment of the sick were conspicuously lacking.

CHAPTER IV

SYSTEMATIZED GROSS PATHOLOGIC
ANATOMY

THUS, as we have seen, Benivieni had recorded a short series of correlated clinical
and postmortem observations at the end of the
fifteenth century, and "Centuries" of cases had
been gathered by Bartholinus, Amatus Lusitanus
and others in the succeeding centuries, works
that included noteworthy individual pathological descriptions and discoveries. No collection of
systematized morbid anatomy was made, however,
until the appearance of the "Sepulchretum anatomicum sive anatomica practica" (1679) of the
Genevan, *Theophilus Bonetus* (1620-89). This
monumental work was well named "a place full
of tombs," as compared to the "Spicilegia" or
"collections of literary scraps" of contemporary
writers. It contained clinical and pathological
descriptions of almost 3000 cases selected from
"the literature" since the time of Hippocrates
(but mostly from the sixteenth and seventeenth
centuries), and is of prime importance in the
history of pathology not only for its intrinsic
worth but as having been the immediate inspiration of the "De sedibus" of Morgagni. Its systematic arrangement, wealth of detail, and its
careful references and indexing make it a happy
hunting ground for early descriptions of pathologic conditions. The great Haller thought it
worth an entire pathological library, as indeed
it almost was, up to 1679. The cases are arranged

in the anatomical order first seen in the Smith
papyrus (head, thorax, etc.) subdivided according to symptoms. Thus the first 130 observations,
occupying 77 pages of my 1700 edition, are on
various kinds of headaches, associated with a
variety of cerebral, meningeal, bony and humoral changes, epilepsy, wounds, tumors and so
on. These are correlated with the postmortem
findings in copious profusion, though some of
the descriptions, to be sure, leave the conditions
either unrecognizable today or requiring considerable interpretation. The author makes numerous comments but modestly abstains from
drawing any extensive conclusions. A greater
boldness or ability to generalize might have
placed him on a par with Morgagni.

Phthisis and "tabes" of glands and bones are
grouped together in a chapter, among the cases
of which is a description of miliary tuberculosis
(Case 17, quoted from Heurnius), "totum parenchyma [pulmonis] minimis tuberculis . . .
oppletum erat." Pneumonia, on the other hand,
fares little better than in the hands of Hippocrates or Soranus and is still confused with
peripneumonia. Among the circulatory diseases
are included Lower's case of tricuspid endocarditis (also Lower's experimental production
of edema [see Chapter VII]), a ruptured aortic
aneurysm described by Marchetti, also syphilis
and tumors of bones, dropsy with obstruction
of veins by abdominal tumors, nephritis chiefly
from ascending infection. A clear description,
perhaps the first, of a cyst of the pituitary gland
is found in Observation 46 of the first section:
A girl of twelve, fat and of a pituitous tempera-

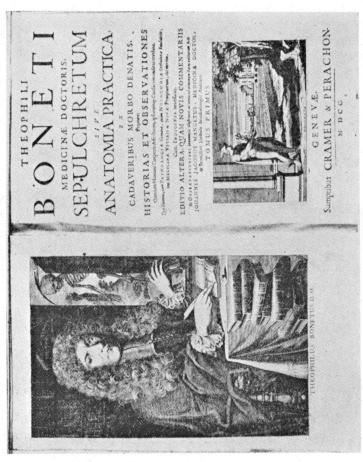

Fig. 6. Theophilus Bonetus. (Portrait from his "Sepulchretum" with title page of a late edition.)

[55]

ment, suffered four months from severe head-
ache until death put an end to her pains and
miseries. At autopsy, no cause could be found
until the surgeon broke with his finger an "abscess adhering to the infundibulum, from which
2 pints of very clear water gushed forth like a
fountain."

Apoplexy, the second symptom treated, includes 76 cases, due not only to hemorrhage into
the brain and on the meninges (quoting Wepfer,
Borelli and others) but also to wounds, abscesses,
viscid humors (!), thrombosis of vessels, frac-
tured skull, and other lesions. In fact, so many
causes are given that we must recognize that the
term is used to include almost any sudden loss
of consciousness without fits.* Observation 13
copies the famous report by Baglivi on the autopsy of his master, Malpighi, who died of a
stroke in spite of bloodletting, scarification, mus-
tard plasters and other remedies. The autopsy
notes of this case, which in vivid conciseness
resemble some of Osler's Blockley records,
showed 2 pounds (?) of black blood in the right
ventricle, though the paralysis was on the right
side, and 6 ounces of yellowish fluid in the left
ventricle. In addition, there was hypertrophy and
dilatation of the left ventricle, atrophy of the
right kidney with dilatation of the pelvis attributed to calculi found in the bladder. "The
remaining viscera were normal."

Between Bonet and Morgagni, three Dutch
pathological collections are to be noted. *Theodor*

* Charles II of England was said to have died of apoplexy
because he had "fits." From the autopsy record, his death appears
to have been due to uremia and certainly not to cerebral hemorrhage.

Kerckring (1640-93) in 1670 published his "Spicilegium anatomicum," containing only about a hundred clinico-pathological observations, but all his own. Of greatest interest to the pathologist perhaps is his recognition, for the first time, that the so-called "polyps of the heart" of practically all the previous observers (see Tulp's illustration) were in reality postmortem clots. *Steven Blankaart's* (1650-1702) "Anatomia practica" was a similar record of about 200 autopsies. Chiari commends his observations on wounds, tuberculosis, uterine cancer and ovarian cysts. The "Thesauri anatomici" (1701-16) of *Frederik Ruysch* (1638-1731) is almost as important in the history of pathologic as of anatomic illustration. His famous museum at Leyden, bought by Peter the Great for 30,000 florins and said to be still visible at Leningrad, contained morbid as well as normal anatomical specimens. Bone lesions, calculi, tumors and cirrhotic livers figure prominently in his "Observationum anatomico chirurgicarum centuria" (1691-1737).

In Italian pathology between Malpighi and Morgagni, the Roman, *Giovanni Maria Lancisi* (1654-1720) alone stands out. In his "De subitaneis mortis" (1707), composed to explain the many sudden deaths of the previous year, he offered cardiac hypertrophy and dilatation as one such cause and noted acute and chronic changes in the valves. France contributed especially to knowledge of the heart in this period. *Raymond de Vieussens* (1641-1716), of Montpellier and Paris, in his treatises of 1706 and 1715 not only gave good postmortem pictures of mitral stenosis and aortic insufficiency, but correlated them with the clinical picture and resultant cardiac dilatation. Even better comprehension of cardiac disease is shown in the next generation in *J. B. Senac's* (1693-1770) "Traité de la structure du coeur, etc." (1749), while his protégé, *Joseph Lieutaud* (1703-80), of Aix en Provence, published in 1767 the leading French pathological collection of the century. This "Historia anatomica-medica," based on 1200 autopsies at the Versailles hospital, as well as on the customary crop from the writings of others, was the first to present the material on the basis of the organ chiefly involved rather than on the symptom. Like Bonetus', a useful record, it is not to be compared with the contemporary "De sedibus" of Morgagni.

Unquestionably one of the greatest figures in the whole history of pathology was *Giovanni Battista Morgagni* (1682-1771), who though he modestly regarded his masterpiece as merely a continuation of Bonetus' work, in reality initiated the scientific study of gross morbid anatomy, by collecting a vast amount of pathologic material, always closely correlated with clinical findings, and arranging and analyzing it in a systematic manner that permitted logical and far-reaching deductions as to the nature of the disease in question and of disease in general. Benivieni, Kerckring, Blankaart, Bonetus and others, as we have seen, had made intelligent but usually short and disconnected post-mortem studies without much systematic sequence. But just as Harvey's glory is in no way dimmed by the notable, even necessary, work of his prede-

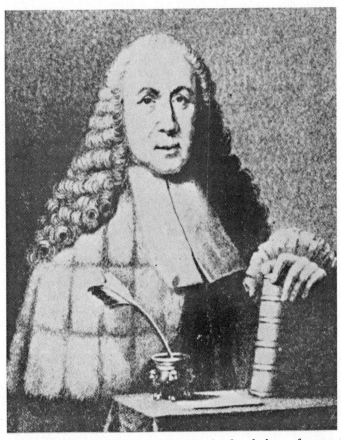

FIG. 7. Giovanni Battista Morgagni, the father of gross
pathology.

cessors, so Morgagni's by its very size, intelligence
of interpretation and thoroughness of method
may be regarded as establishing the anatomic
concept in nosology and as placing pathologic
anatomy on a scientific basis as a branch of
modern medicine.

Born at Forli, Morgagni at the age of fourteen showed a precocious ability to write prose
and poetry and to discuss philosophic texts in
public. At sixteen, he entered the University of
Bologna, where he became a pupil of Malpighi's
pupil, Valsalva, to whom he owed and acknowl-
edged much. At twenty-four he published his
first book, "Adversaria anatomica," containing
noteworthy anatomical studies, which was followed by a second series of "Adversaria" and
numerous "Epistolae anatomicae." At twenty-
nine he was called to the chair of theoretic
medicine at Padua, and to that of anatomy
four years later—a chair which during 200 years
was held by the matchless succession of Vesalius,
Realdus Columbus, Fabricius of Aquapendente,
Spigelius, Marchetti, Valsalva and Morgagni.
As they all contributed to morbid as well as
normal anatomy, we can properly include them
in a pathological list of honor. At Padua, Morgagni taught and studied for fifty-six years, the
last of the great Italians to be a medical focus
for the civilized world. At the ripe age of seventy-
nine he published his last and greatest work,
"De sedibus et causis morborum per anatomen
indigatis" (1761), as a series of letters to a
friend, which in some 700 case and autopsy reports, performed by himself or his associates,
covered practically every phase of pathological

anatomy approachable with the naked eye. The five books concern: Diseases of the Head, Thorax, Abdomen, Surgical Diseases or those involving the whole body, and Addenda. Besides emphasizing the need for clinical facts in a given case and clinical knowledge on the part of the pathologist, in this monumental work Morgagni placed on a firm basis a careful and thorough autopsy technique based on a mastery of normal anatomy and designed to throw light not only on the cause of death but on the cause of the disease and its various manifestations. Mistakes, to be sure, were there aplenty; cause was mistaken for effect, related phenomena, such as tumor metastases, were observed but not connected, the unimportant stressed and the important neglected, even some false observations were made; but these may well be lost sight of in the mass of important additions to existing knowledge.

To consider one system as a sample, in the cardiovascular system he observed: the structural changes in a case of angina pectoris, the first reported case of heart block with Adams-Stokes' syndrome, vegetative endocarditis (including one that complicated an acute gonorrhea), the two causes of apoplexy (cerebral softening and hemorrhage from hardened vessels) and the production of paralysis on the opposite side of the body from the cerebral lesion, and, like Harvey, a case of rupture of the heart. His knowledge of aneurysms was accurate (see 3 cases of Long's "Readings") and he apparently believed in their frequent association with lues venerea, though he made no direct statement to that effect. He was of course familiar with syphilis of the skin, knew its ravages in the bones and described gummata of the liver and brain (the latter a first description).

The nature of pneumonia, with its change of the lung tissue "to have the substance of liver" (i.e., hepatization), was for the first time made clear. The possibilities of different histories and lesions of tuberculosis were recognized (see 2 cases in Long's "Readings"), though autopsies on the tuberculous as a rule and at least one case of anthrax were avoided. One must at times read with extra care to realize the true significance of the descriptions. Typhoid fever (intestinal ulcers, splenic tumor and enlarged mesenteric glands), blenorrhagia, cirrhosis, and acute yellow atrophy, renal calculi, tuberculosis, atrophy and hydronephrosis, neoplasms of the esophagus, stomach, pylorus, rectum, pancreas, ovary, adrenal ("ren succenturiatus") and liver are among those described. Morgagni apparently had not mastered the concept of metatasis, which was to baffle pathologists for another century. Cerebral abscess he showed to be due to and not the cause of ear discharges.

After Morgagni in Italy, his successor *Caldani* was chiefly concerned in harmonizing his master's views with the doctrines of his favorite, Haller, while *Antonio Scarpa* (1747-1832), the master's most celebrated pupil, was more distinguished for his anatomical discoveries and artistic illustration of his own works than for his pathological contributions (hernia, diseases of the eye and bones, internal lesions in arteriosclerosis, true and false aneurysms).

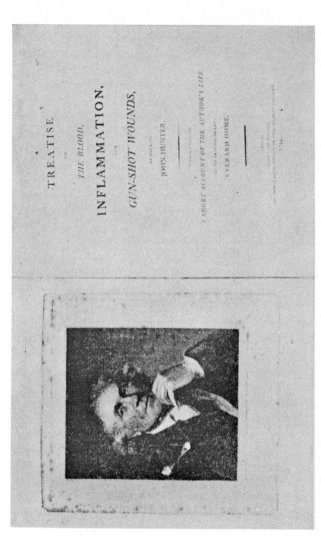

FIG. 8. John Hunter. (From an engraving after Reynolds' painting, with title page of his "Treatise on the Blood, Inflammation and Gunshot Wounds.")

In Holland, *Edward Sandifort* (1742-1814) carried on the tradition of anatomic museums and atlases. His "Observationes anatomicae-pathologicae" (1777-81) and "Museum . . . Descriptum" (1793-1835) beautifully illustrate the contents of the Leyden museum with such specimens as congenital lesions of the heart and other viscera, hernias and intestinal obstructions, bony ankyloses and inflammations, ulcerative endocarditis and so on.

The kind of material that Bonetus and Morgagni gathered for their books was being collected by the Hunters in England for their teaching and their museums.* Though the elder, *William Hunter* (1718-83), was more concerned with anatomy and obstetrics, his teaching at the famous Great Windmill Street School included morbid anatomy, while his accumulation of specimens of all kinds is preserved for posterity in the celebrated Hunterian Museum at Glasgow. His greater younger brother, *John Hunter* (1728-93), rightly regarded as one of the leading lights of British medicine, also accumulated a great museum of some 13,000 specimens, now the Hunterian Museum of the College of Surgeons in London. His experimental achievements will be considered in the last chapter.

The current of pathological thought received an important addition from the Hunters' nephew, *Matthew Baillie* (1761-1823), last and most eminent of the holders of the famous Gold Headed Cane. His book on "The Morbid Anat-

* See d'Arcy Power's "Medicine in the British Isles" in this Series.

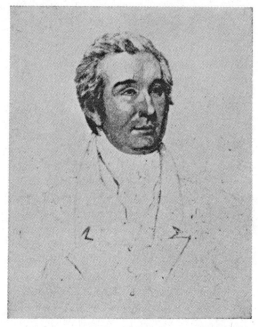

FIG. 9. Matthew Baillie. (From an unfinished stipple
engraving.)

omy of Some of the Most Important Parts of
the Human Body" (1793), was the first systematic text on pathological anatomy in any
language. Though brief and not covering the
entire body, it described in simple, clear language the lesions that the several organs and
systems were prone to, much as in the special
pathology sections of modern textbooks. Case
reports were not included, though they were
added in the German translation; in other words,
pathology was now treated for the first time as
an independent science. The success of the book
was prompt: a second and larger edition appeared in 1797 (here rheumatism of the heart
was for the first time mentioned in print) and
a supplementary atlas, also the first of its kind,
was published from 1799-1802. This had appeared in ten fasciculi, each containing eight
fine plates of several figures each, engraved on
steel after drawings by William Clift, with a
liberal explanatory text. The sequence is the
same as in the twenty-four chapters; namely,
cardiovascular system, respiratory, digestive,
genitourinary, brain and meninges. The artistic
engravings are too numerous to mention (it was
the hey-day of the steel plate) but many of the
illustrations, such as those of acute and chronic
aortic valvulitis, hepatic cirrhosis (called tubercle), had to await proper interpretation in the
light of better pathologic knowledge. The pictures of an ovarian teratoma and a hydatidiform mole are famous. Baillie's work was translated into German by Soemmerring and also into
French and Italian, and set the mode for similar

works by Vogel (1804), Meckel (1812), Otto (1814) and Cruveilhier (1816).

Baillie, after receiving a good classical education at Balliol, assisted his uncles, the Hunters, and later took over with Cruikshank the famous Great Windmill Street School of Anatomy. It was there that he gathered material for his book and his atlas illustrations. He was one of the first to describe transposition of the viscera (1788) and dermoid cysts of the ovary (1789).

Thus by the end of the eighteenth century we find gross pathologic anatomy established as a firm basis for medical science; chiefly by the vast number of Morgagni's observations, on the whole well correlated with clinical records, and a beginning made with Baillie's text of systematic treatment of the subject as an independent discipline. Though, as we have seen, theoretic systems still held sway in academic pedagogy, the way for Bichat's study of the tissues, Rokitansky's gross descriptions, and Virchow's cellular pathology had been definitely opened.

CHAPTER V

PATHOLOGIC ANATOMY OF THE TIS-SUES AND PRE-CELLULAR PATHOLOGY

MARIE-FRANCOIS-XAVIER BICHAT (1771-1802), as well as being known as the father of histology, may justly be ranked with Morgagni and Virchow as one of the founders of modern pathology, though his contribution is perhaps more elusive than are those of the other two. It is true that man's organism as a whole had long been a subject of scrutiny and an imposing edifice of knowledge of the lesions of separate organs had been slowly rising for over two centuries; but a new concept was needed to pave the way for the triumphs of modern pathology. This Bichat supplied for morbid as well as for normal anatomy by his presentation of the various tissues as units—hence the word "histology" ($\iota\sigma\tau\delta s$ —a tissue), a term which has only gradually and indirectly acquired the connotation, "microscopic." Bichat's work was accomplished in the short thirty-one years of an existence handicapped by tuberculosis, and, strangely enough at first sight, without the aid of the microscope that had already served biologists for over a century. His methods were those of dissection and of treating his material with "various chemical reagents as heat, air, water, acids, alkalies, salts, desiccation, maceration, putrefaction, boiling, etc., fixing with precision the limits of each organized tissue." To be sure, he had had forerunners, such as his mas-

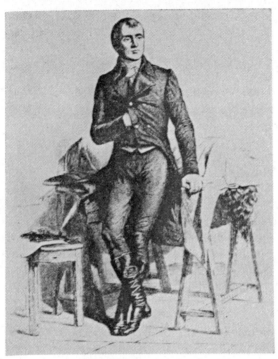

FIG. 10. Marie-Francois-Xavier Bichat.
(From an old engraving.)

ter Pinel and Andreas Bonn of Amsterdam, whose Leyden dissertation, "De continuationibus membranorum" (1763), foreshadows much of the anatomic side of Bichat's tissue concepts. But to Bichat we owe the great step of establishing tissues rather than organs as the important biological unit. Without the aid of a good microscope further basic progress was impossible at the moment.

Though most of Bichat's published works bear anatomical titles, he was well aware of their significance for disease: "The more we examine bodies, the more we must be convinced of the necessity of considering local disease not from the standpoint of the compound organs, which are rarely affected as a whole, but from the standpoint of their different textures, which are almost always attacked separately." He specifies examples from the meninges, the coats of the eye and the larynx, the three layers of the heart, and so on. One has but to think also of such further examples as the selective affinity of intestinal typhoid lesions for Peyer's patches, of various bacteria for the heart valves, of tetanus toxin for the nervous system, and still unexplored selectivities of cancer metastasis, to ascribe an importance to this concept that makes it second only to that of Cellular Pathology itself. He distinguished twenty-one kinds of tissues: nervous, connective (which he called "cellular" in the gross sense of acquiring spaces or cells when inflated), vascular, muscular, osseous, cartilaginous, mucous, serous, synovial, absorbent, glandular, dermoid, etc. These were looked on as the elementary structures which combined to make up organs, the units of specific functions. Each of the tissues had its characteristic vital property in the Stahlian sense, disease consisting of the weakening of this vital property to a point where it was unable to cope with harmful forces introduced from the exterior. He divided morbid anatomy into two parts: (1) the alterations common to each system wherever located (i.e., our general pathology) and (2) diseases peculiar to each region (i.e., our special pathology). Disease of a tissue is essentially the same, no matter in what organ the involved tissue may be. If a few more years had been spared him, a book on pathology would doubtless have been forthcoming, as Bichat was well aware of the advantages to be gained by postmortem examination and gave his last course of lectures on pathologic anatomy. Though these are preserved for us in Béclard's transcription, they can in no sense be taken as representing Bichat's complete views on or knowledge of the subject. The original editions of his chief works: the "Traité des membranes" (1799-1800), "Anatomie descriptive" (1801-03) and "Anatomie générale" (1802), are obviously of great historical importance, and yet, strange to say, they are still purchasable for very modest sums.

For the furtherance of the tissue concept we must look to Cruveilhier in France and to Johannes Müller and his pupil, Jacob Henle, in Germany, all of whom appeared on the scene enough later to take advantage also of the recently introduced Cell Theory. Bichat's concept had been sufficiently well established, however, to constitute a large factor in many of the im-

portant discoveries that were to be made in
France and England in the succeeding generation.

With the French Revolution, whether producing it or produced by it, there flourished a generation of outstanding Frenchmen, unsurpassed
anywhere for that period. French medicine led
the world, just as its political and military genius
for years successfully withstood the rest of Europe. Even the Englishman, Forbes, the trans-
lator of Laënnec, speaks of the "great superiority
of French pathologists." Led by *J. N. Corvisart*
(1755-1821), the rediscoverer of percussion, and
Ph. Pinel (1745-1826), the initiator of the modern treatment of the insane, the French school
was dominant, even over the great Anglo-Irish
school of that period, until superseded by the
German pathologists, bacteriologists and student clinicians of the latter half of the nineteenth century. Pinel's "Nosographie philoso-
phique" (1789), which went through many editions in the next quarter century, had paved the
way for Bichat, not by its exaggerated subdivisions of diseases, but by its tendency to show
similarity in disorders of similar tissues, of which
he considered five. Pleuritis, henceforth, meant,
as its name indicates, inflammation of the pleura,
and not the vague jumble of either lung or
pleura disorder, or both, that had hitherto maintained. The fundamental influence of the work
of Pinel's pupil, Bichat, was apparent henceforth on both sides of the Channel.

Corvisart's book "Les maladies et les lesions
organiques du coeur et gros vaisseaux" (1806),
the greatest on the heart since Senac's, likewise

developed his topic from the point of view of the different tissues of the heart, rather than of the heart as an organ. Incidentally, on the much discussed item of heart polyps, though he stated that most were antemortem, he obviously had good criteria for the differentiation of ante-mortem from postmortem clots. He was twice wrong on syphilis, which he on the one hand regarded as an important cause of all valvular lesions, and on the other failed to connect with aortic aneurysms, about which he wrote exten-sively. These were details, however, that can well be disregarded in favor of his great service in establishing frequent postmortem examinations as a means of tracing the development of disease as well as its end changes, and in fostering great pupils, headed by Bayle and the immortal Laën-nec.

Next in the flood of important French works was the Provencal, *Gaspard-Laurent Bayle's* (1774-1816) "Recherches sur la phthisie pul-monaire" (1810),* a disease which accounted for one-fifth to one-fourth of all deaths at that time. Bayle recognized six kinds of phthisis, a term which then included any progressive degen-eration of the lung attended with emaciation, of which the commonest type was correctly desig-nated tuberculosis. He gave the best description of the varieties of tubercle to date, though none too good at that. His "granular" type we may recognize as miliary tuberculosis (which he was among the first to describe, though he described it as cartilaginous in nature), and "calculous"

* For this and subsequent works on the subject see Gerald Webb's volume on "Tuberculosis" in this Series.

as calcified tubercles; while the "melanotic" indicated both melanoma and anthracotic fibrosis,
and the "cancerous" was correctly regarded. The
"ulcerous" variety included a mixture of abscess, gangrene, bronchiectasis and unrecognized
tuberculosis. He successfully correlated tuberculosis of the lung with the same disease in other
organs and upheld its position as an independent
disease rather than as a mere sequel of a variety
of diseases. He obviously recognized tuberculous
meningitis (Obs. 8), a discovery that is often
attributed to Papavoine (1830).

A man of far greater importance to pathology,
as well as being "the greatest clinician of all
time," was *Réné Théophile Hyacinthe Laënnec*
(1781-1826), like Bayle, an early victim of the
disease that he so greatly illuminated. Coming
from his native Brittany, he studied at the
Charité under Corvisart, Bayle, and also with
Bichat and Dupuytren (what an opportunity!).
When only twenty-two, the year before he received his doctorate, he was already giving a
course of lectures on pathologic anatomy. After
his death, a Preface to a textbook on pathologic
anatomy that he never had opportunity to finish
was found among his papers and later published
(1884). His pathologic studies, unremittingly
followed throughout his short life, were as necessary as his mastery of percussion and his own discovery, mediate auscultation, in founding the
art of physical diagnosis and in unravelling the
many mysteries of pulmonary pathology. He
constantly practiced his belief that diseases cannot be more certainly distinguished than by their
anatomical characters. Most of his discoveries are

to be found in his great book on "Mediate Auscultation," of which the first edition was published in 1819, two short years after his discovery
of the stethoscope. The second enlarged edition
("Treatise on Diseases of the Chest"), which
appeared in 1826, the year of his death, gives
not only the various physical signs elicited in
the chest, as in the first edition, but also the
pathologic anatomy, diagnosis and treatment of
each disease encountered. Of several, such as
bronchiectasis, emphysema, pulmonary apoplexy
(infarct), hemorrhagic pleurisy, pneumothorax,
melanoma, he was the virtual, if not the actual,
discoverer. In the case of emphysema, for example, occasional large lungs had been noted
since the time of Bonetus, and Baillie had noted
their failure to collapse, their occasional huge
projecting alveoli, and even subpleural extrav-
asation; but any comparison of the written accounts at once makes it apparent that true comprehension of the disease was first acquired by
Laënnec. The pathology of phthisis occupies,
in Forbes' translation, over sixty pages of vividly
clear description, most of which still holds.
Laënnec correctly differentiated Bayle's non-tu-
berculous types of phthisis, and, with the insight
of genius, followed the tubercle through its gray,
yellow and conglomerate varieties to the development of excavations and "encysted" forms. His
"jelly like tuberculous infiltration" we may assume to be our gelatinous (tuberculous) pneumonia. When we consider that the microscope (a
pre-achromatic affair applied to unstained tissues) was rarely used by him (as in determining
the size of emphysematous alveoli), these de-

scriptions invoke one's greatest admiration. Laënnec correctly upheld Bayle's view that tuberculosis was a direct product of inflammation and
not secondary to other conditions; but his pes-
simism appears in the remark, "the real cause,
like that of all disease, being probably beyond
our reach." By the irony of fate, his name remains attached, not to any of his great discoveries, but to a chance, brief consideration of
the hob-nailed liver which had been recognized
since the days of Hippocrates. On account of the
yellow color of the granular indurations, he proposed the name "cirrhosis" (κιῤῥός, yellow).
This appears in all editions of his great work in
the section on chronic pleurisy, as a footnote to
the description of a case that presented both conditions at autopsy.

Following Laënnec's truly epoch-making work,
post-mortem examinations and the new art of
physical diagnosis rapidly became the rage. In
1826, the year of Laënnec's second edition, appeared *Pierre Bretonneau's* (1771-1862) important monograph on "Diphthérite," (his own
term) definitely establishing the disease diphtheria and its identity with croup and malignant
angina, a question that had remained obscure
since the days of Aretaeus. Before the discovery of
the achromatic lens, he was using the microscope
to determine such details as ecchymoses and fol-
licular orifices. Bretonneau previously (1820)
had observed the lesions in Peyer's patches in
cases of continued fever, soon to be recognized as
typhoid. In fact, this term was proposed in Louis'
work on gastroenteritis the same year (1829)
that Bretonneau's article on *dothienentérite* ap-

peared. At last a breach was appearing in the hitherto mysterious and impregnable wall of the continued fevers!

The importance of continued fever had for centuries demanded classifications and reclassifications, but always on the basis of symptoms. At this very moment, in France, *F. J. V. Broussais* (1772-1838) was proposing an anatomical, albeit speculative and incorrect, basis for fever that proceeded from the Brunonian theory of irritation. Requiring a local site of the febrile irritation and in spite of a laudable regard for autopsies, he fixed on "gastroenteritis" as the basis of all pathology, and met the situation for his patients with universal starving and leeching, i.e., depletion ("Histoire sur phlegmasies," 1808). Fantastical as this may seem today, for years it held sway in the face of contrary evidence; neither was it the last of hypothetical theories of disease to carry great weight, Cruveilhier's phlebitis and Rokitansky's dyscrases were still to come.

Fortunately for long-suffering humanity, a master of objective observation and statistical analysis now appeared, one who agreed with Rousseau that "the truth is in the facts and not in my opinion that estimates them." *P. C. A. Louis* (1787-1872) devoted his life to careful studies in the wards and postmortem rooms of the great Paris hospitals, the Pitié, the Charité and the Hôtel Dieu; and incidentally he exerted an important influence on medicine in this country. Since the fostering guidance of the Edinburgh school—and through it, of Boerhaave—no external stimulus has had a greater effect on American medical science than Louis' training

of such men as Gerhard, Pennock and Stillé in
Philadelphia and Holmes, the Jacksons and Shat-
tucks in Boston. His statistical method has ever
since held a basic position as one of the exact
instruments of medical investigation. First of
his important works was a study of phthisis
(1825), based on 358 autopsies and 1960 clinical cases.

Of even greater importance to medical science
was his "Recherches . . . sur la maladie connue
sous les noms de fièvre typhoide, putride,
adynamique" (1829). Based on an analysis of
138 cases of typhoid with 50 autopsies (in *all* of
which the characteristic changes in the ileum
were present) compared to 83 other fatal acute
fevers, this for all time established the pathologic picture of typhoid fever. It only remained
to differentiate it from the other important continued fever, typhus, with which it had the common symptom of stupor (τῦφος). Huxham's
differentiation of the "putrid malignant"
(typhus) from the "slow nervous" fever (usually
typhoid) indicates that this difference had already been sensed. Garrison quotes descriptions
of epidemics of each variety by Hufeland and of
typhoid with autopsies by Roederer and Wagler
(1762); but here as elsewhere the disease was
confused with intermittent and other continued
fevers, such as dysentery.

The distinction between the two fevers was
finally demonstrated by *W. W. Gerhard* (1809-
72), Louis' most distinguished pupil, who in the
wards and deadhouses of the Philadelphia and
Pennsylvania Hospitals brought out the fundamental differences of a Philadelphia epidemic

of typhus fever (1836) from the disease described by his master. In but one of some 50 cases autopsied was any change found in the "glands of Peyer, and in that only a little reddened and thickened"; the characteristic typhoid changes in the spleen and mesenteric nodes were also absent.

Space forbids more than mere mention of such French leaders as Chomel, Portal, Piorry and Andral, whose "Essai d'hématologie pathologique" (1843) was a pioneer in emphasizing the chemical study of the blood in disease. Bouillaud, Broussais' successor in pitiless bleeding, is usually credited with correlating heart disease with rheumatic fever (1836); but this connection had been common knowledge in England for more than a generation (Wells, 1810; Hawkins' Gulstonian Lectures, 1826, etc.). It was apparently first described in Pitcairn's Lectures (1788) and promulgated in Baillie's second edition (1797).

Two more French achievements remain to be described: the creation of two of the earliest independent chairs of pathologic anatomy (see Appendix). The first to be established anywhere was that of the then French University of Strasbourg, where *J. F. Lobstein* (1777-1835), of Giessen but long resident in Strasbourg, was established in 1819 on the recommendation of the great Cuvier. Lobstein's "Traité d'anatomie pathologique" (Paris, 1829), of which unfortunately the part on special pathology was never written, is of interest both for its historical review of the subject from the Pharaohs to Corvisart and for the advance that

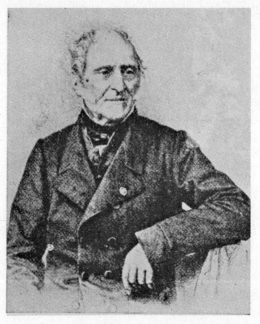

FIG. 11A. Jean Cruveilhier (portrait in older life).

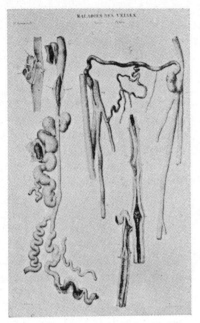

FIG. 11B. Illustration from Cruveilhier's atlas.

it records over Gaub's standard work of the preceding half century. The book was conceived in the spirit that "it is not the dead organ that medicine wishes to understand, but the living organ, exercising the functions peculiar to it." It had the threefold aid of clear pathologic description, comprehension of the pathogenesis (a term coined by Lobstein) and correlation of morbid anatomy with symptoms, and it also emphasized the need for animal experimentation.

In 1836, at the suggestion of the surgeon Dupuytren, there was established (1836) the year after his death a chair of pathological anatomy in the University of Paris. Its first occupant was *Jean Cruveilhier* (1791-1873), who twenty years before, the year of his graduation, had written an "Essai sur l'anatomie pathologique" (1816) in several volumes. This rather immature collection recognized the work of Baillie, Bichat and his colleagues, Bayle and Laënnec, but made no pretense at being a complete presentation. One finds in it but little of his theory that all organic changes are due to morbid secretions into the interstitial tissues from the all powerful capillaries, a doctrine that was so prominent in his "Traité de l'anatomie pathologique générale" (5 vols., 1849-1864) (see later chapter on Inflammation). More valuable today is his splendid "Atlas d'anatomie pathologique" (1835-42), beautifully lithographed, but restricted entirely to gross preparations. Its 240 folio plates, many in color and all accompanied by copious text (originally issued in forty separate parts over a period of seven years) make it unquestionably the greatest work of its kind ever published. One could dilate on numerous cancers, excellently portrayed and described, on Siamese twins carefully dissected, multiple erectile angiomata, and so on almost *ad infinitum*; but these volumes must be seen to be appreciated.

Across the Channel, nineteenth century medicine advanced less boldly. Baillie's book, to be sure, was widely known and Bichat's emphasis on tissues rather than organs had its influence there. A few important observations, such as the recognition of rheumatism of the heart, just mentioned, are to be recorded. The most important of these were contained in the treatise by the Birmingham surgeon, *Joseph Hodgson* (1788-1869), "On the Diseases of Arteries and Veins" (1815). This not only gave the best illustrations of aneurysms of various kinds that had thus far been published, but also excellent illustrations of aortic valvular endocarditis (one fungating and perforated, one chronic) and what is said to be the first description of aneurysmal dilatation of the aortic arch. The work so impressed the French, to whom it owed little, that they spoke of aortic aneurysm as the *maladie d'Hodgson*.

Other important English pathological publications of the time were those splendid pioneers among pathological Atlases, "The Principles and Illustrations of Morbid Anatomy" (1834) by *James Hope* (1801-41) and the "Illustrations of the Elementary Forms of Disease" (1838) by *(Sir) Robert Carswell* (1793-1857). Following Cruveilhier's first *livraisons* by only a few years, their brilliantly colored lithographs, each drawn "from nature" by the author himself, opened a new vision of gross pathology to British medical eyes. Carswell's is the better of the two, though not the equal either in scope or execution of Cruveilhier's magnificent folios. The accompanying texts at times reflect a strangely antique pathology: In Carswell's atlas, for instance, secondary cancer nodules in the liver were regarded as local changes of liver tissue brought about by the cancerous humor in the blood; such diverse lesions as thrombi, angiomata, adhesions, cysts, ichthyosis, etc., are grouped under the vague term, "analogous tissues"; "softening" apparently included infarcts, anemic states, postmortem autolysis and other unrecognizable conditions. His final section on tubercle, however, profited by Laënnec's views and gave pictures that easily surpass Laënnec's in their fidelity to nature. Carswell, a Paisleyan graduate of Aberdeen, who had been made Professor of Morbid Anatomy at the University College, London, in 1831 (see Appendix), wrote well on multiple sclerosis, recognized the atrophic element in pulmonary emphysema and was one of the leading English pathologists of his generation.

With the spread of Laënnec's doctrine in the second quarter of the century the English were quick to follow the lead of the new developments in France. Especially were "the great men of Guy's" successful in applying English common sense and originality to the newly opened and fallow fields of correlated bedside and postmortem room observation. Most illustrious of the group was *Richard Bright* (1789-1858), immortalized by his description of chronic non-suppurative nephritis, still best known as "Bright's disease." It must be noted, however, that his useful contributions were by no means limited to the kidney: numerous are his shrewd observations on pancreatic diabetes and diabetic steatorrhea (1832), acute yellow atrophy (1836), Jacksonian epilepsy (1836), status lymphaticus (1838), ovarian tumors, echinococcus cysts. In his "Reports of Medical Cases" (1827) he correctly differentiated renal from cardiac, hepatic and other types of dropsy, and was the first to correlate this and the previously observed albuminuria with the nephritic changes observed at autopsy. The first 23 cases reported, mostly with a *sectio cadaveris* and beautifully illustrated, establish a definite clinico-pathologic picture. His "large white" and "red (with hematuria) kidneys" of acutely fatal cases were terms persisting till our own student days; while for his three developmental stages of mottled flabbiness, enlargement with cortical granulation and interstitial deposit and finally a hard contracted kidney, modern terminology might find some grounds for substituting "simple nephrosis," "early and late chronic glomerulonephritis." Without the microscopic and selectively stained thin sections, he was spared the refinements of modern classifications of renal disease. Those who look on biochemistry as one of the youngest of the medical sciences should be surprised to learn of the antiquity of determinations of blood urea, which were well known to Bright in correlation with uremia, as well as the hyperglycemia of diabetes, observed by his associate, *George Rees* (1813-89).

Associated with Bright for many years as physician to Guy's Hospital was *Thomas Addison* (1793-1860), fated to be known by his contemporaries as an eminently practical clinician and diagnostician, and to write in older life a short treatise of thirty odd pages that made him immortal. In his monograph "On the Constitutional and Local Effects of Disease of the Supra-Renal Capsules" (1855), an expansion of an article written six years earlier, he not only gave the clinical and pathologic picture of the disease of these glands that we now know as Addison's disease, but also described "a very remarkable form of general anemia," the disease pernicious anemia to which Trousseau later gave the name Addisonian anemia. Necessarily in ignorance of the various cells to be found in the blood and of their relation to spleen and bone marrow and almost without the resources of the microscope* and of cellular pathology, he naturally failed to discover any organic lesion that would serve adequately as the cause of the anemia. As a matter of fact, this knowledge is still lacking, and it is only in the past decade that real knowledge of the mechanism of this disease has been forthcoming. The 11 cases included in the monograph all showed marked suprarenal disease (4 being tuberculous, 3 cancerous and 1 apparently apoplectic). This work and Claude Bernard's discovery of the glycogen-storing function of the liver have been properly

---

* In one case a portion of the semilunar ganglion and solar plexus was, like the heart, "pronounced" as the result of microscopic examination to have undergone fatty degeneration.

regarded as the most significant starters of the now all-important study of endocrinology.

The pathologist to Guy's Hospital, *Thomas Hodgkin* (1798-1866) also contributed his share of English pathologic discoveries. He correctly described aortic valvular insufficiency three years before Corrigan, with whose name the condition is usually connected. In 1832, his first paper in the *Medico Chirurgical Transactions,* "On Some Morbid Appearances of the Absorbent Glands and the Spleen," described the clinical and pathologic changes of the disease, now called "lymphogranuloma," or "Hodgkin's disease" (so named by Wilks, 1865). The 7 cases included in this report are now believed to have included leucemia and tuberculosis of the lymphoid tissues; but most were true examples of Hodgkin's disease. Some of his original specimens are still extant in Guy's Museum and have yielded excellent histological details to modern technical preparation.. Hodgkin's study, of course, was confined to gross observations, the histological picture of the disease not being established till the end of the century by Sternberg and Dorothy Reed. His "Lectures on the Morbid Anatomy of the Serous and Mucous Membranes" (1836-40) were more appreciated in his day, constituting an important English development of tissue pathology.

Laënnec's influence was reflected in Ireland by that brilliant group whose chief members were *Abraham Colles, John Cheyne, Robert Adams, R. J. Graves, Dominic Corrigan* and *William Stokes.* In the field of morbid anatomy, their chief contribution was Corrigan's descrip-

tion of aortic valve insufficiency (1832), which
he illustrated and correlated with the water-
hammer pulse of that disease (Corrigan's pulse).
In the broader aspects of pathology, the group
is noted for the descriptions of Cheyne-Stokes'
respiration, Adams-Stokes' syndrome (heart-
block), exophthalmic goiter (Graves' disease)
and many other shrewd observations of abnormal
function. Invaluable and original as were these
British contributions, one has but to glance
through their publications to see how much their
authors felt that they owed to their French colleagues.

   Carl Rokitansky (1804-78), correctly regarded
with Morgagni as the greatest of all gross descriptive pathologists, presents the curious combination of having made pathological contributions
of the greatest importance and yet of having
promulgated an anachronistic humoral theory
of disease a short decade before the rational
basis of disease change was established by Virchow. Coming to the Allgemeines Krankenhaus
at Vienna as a volunteer under the incompetent
Biermeyer at a time (1824) when pathology was
far from flourishing there, Rokitansky became
Johannes Wagner's (1800-32) assistant in 1828
(see Appendix), was promoted to acting head
on his chief's premature death four years later,
ausserordentlich professor in 1834 and full professor in 1838. With Skoda and Hebra, he soon
became one of the leading lights of the brilliant
Young Viennese School, which was recognized by
Wunderlich as early as 1841 as initiating the
world leadership of German medicine. Deriving
its inspiration largely from France and England,

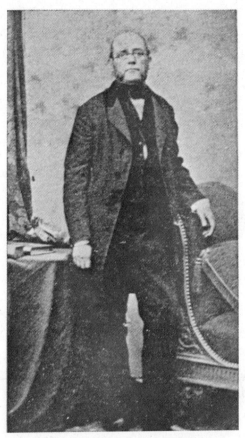

FIG. 12. Karl Rokitansky.
(From an original photograph.)

it produced such prominent figures as Hyrtl, von
Brucke and Pollitzer and a succession of younger
men that have made Vienna a Mecca for medical students to this day. The wealth of pathologic
material that is still available there is to be
traced to Rokitansky, who in his fifty years is said
to have performed over 30,000 autopsies himself
and had material from 60,000 available.

Early influenced by the embryological studies
of *Johann Friedrich Meckel* (1781-1833), Rokitansky throughout his long career paid close attention to anomalies. This culminated in his
great monograph on "Die Defekte der Scheiden-
wände des Herzens" (1875) which achieved the
distinction, seldom reached in the biological sciences, of correctly predicting that certain unob-
served cardiac anomalies would later be discovered. Long before, he had established Meckel's
fundamentally important dictum that most malformations are not the result of mysterious supernatural influence but "represent certain stages
of the development of the embryo and of its
organs" where growth has stopped or continued
abnormally. His great Manual ("Handbuch der
pathologischen Anatomie," 1842-46), far surpassing the previous leaders, Baillie's and Cruveilhier's, is largely classified into anomalies of
number of parts, size, form, position, connection,
color, consistence, texture, contents. General
pathology he regarded as due to anomalies of organization, special pathology to "the special
anomalies of individual textures and organs."
While pathologic anatomy was a local affair,
only indirectly revealing the existence of general disease, disease itself was "referred al-

most without exception to the blood (the fluids) ." This was empirically viewed as an anomaly of admixture or *"crasis"* (built from a supposititious "blastema" or primitive fluid from which cells and tissues were formed) —the unfortunate "monstrous anachronism," which Virchow early demolished. Though Rokitansky foresaw the eventful importance of a then non-existent chemical pathology and stressed the existence of purely local disease (i.e., independent of crasis influence) , yet he soon upheld a dyscrasis for most every important disease or disease group (e.g., typhoid, exanthematous, tuberculous, cancerous, croupous fibrin—alpha, beta and gamma varieties—and so on *ad nauseam*) , further complicated by possible degenerations or by the fantastical culmination of an interconversion of crases. A true scientist, and of "genial and unassuming" disposition, however, he accepted the truth of Virchow's criticisms and the crases disappeared from the later editions of his manual (1855-61) . Virchow, in his Review* of the third edition, recognized this greatness of soul: "How highly must we esteem the man who could forget and learn so much; for whom it was not sufficient to recognize his mistakes but who took the trouble to correct them in the light of the more painstaking, methodical researches of his own pupils." Even in 1895 Virchow regarded the Handbuch as preëminent for the clearness and accuracy of its descriptions and the wealth of its original observations.

To Rokitansky must be allowed the imperishable glory of having permanently established the

* *Wien. med. Wchnschr.,* 5:401,1855.

line of progress begun by Bonetus and Morgagni,
so that diseases thereafter were viewed, not
merely as groups of symptoms and congestions
or other fancied changes, but from the solid
point of view of the underlying structural
changes in the organs concerned. Among his individual contributions to pathology, was the development of a method of performing autopsies,
which with Virchow's method persists in modified form today; also pioneer studies of the more
important diseases of the arteries (1852), the
spondylolisthetic pelvis (1839), intestinal ileus;
and elaborations of the knowledge of emphysema, acute yellow atrophy (which he
named) (1843), perforating gastric ulcer, lardaceous disease, renal and other cysts (see the
plates in his manual showing good cellular detail) and the differentiation between lobar and
lobular pneumonia and between Bright's disease and lardaceous disease of the kidney. Se-
curing an adequate microscope for the first time
in 1842, Rokitansky began careful and successful studies which were incorporated in his later
editions. Firmly convinced to the end of the
prime importance of pathologic anatomy both to
the art of medicine and the science of biology,
he was held in high honor by his contemporaries,
and on his retirement four years before his death
a city-wide testimonial celebration was given
him by the Viennese.

He was succeeded for six years by *Richard
Heschl* (1824-81), after whose death the chair
was occupied by *Hans Kundrat* (1845-93), the
original describer of lymphosarcoma. On the
death of the latter, *Anton Weichselbaum* (1845-

1920), discoverer of the meningococcus, succeeded to the professorship, while *Alexander Kolisko* (1857-1918) took charge of medico-legal pathology and *Richard Paltauf* (1858-1924) became director of the Institute for Pathologic Histology and Bacteriology.

Rokitansky's influence was extended to Prague where his assistant *Hans Chiari* (1851-1916) followed Klebs in 1882 as Professor in the German University. For a quarter century, till his shift to von Recklinghausen's chair at Strasbourg in 1906, Chiari made Prague one of the leading pathologic centers of Europe. His history of pathologic anatomy (in Puschmann's "Handbuch") is a rich source of detailed information.

In clinical fields the new pathologic attitude toward disease was quickly apparent. Skoda's study of percussion and auscultation (1839), like Laënnec's, derived much of its value from close pathologic correlation, just as, to a lesser extent, did Semmelweis' demonstration of the contagiousness of puerperal fever. In surgery, a kindred spirit was added in the person of *Theodor Billroth* (1829-94), a graduate of Berlin, who came to Vienna from Zurich in 1867. For a full quarter century there, he promoted scientific surgery by the study and operative application of the underlying pathological principles (Naunyn's "Autopsies *in vivo*"). Through his numerous prominent pupils, as well as his own achievements, he was of first importance in inaugurating the painstaking and complex surgical procedures that the requisite pathologic knowledge, as well as the newly discovered anesthesia and antisepsis, had made possible.

CHAPTER VI

CELLULAR PATHOLOGY

ONE of the greatest puzzles in the complicated story of the progress of medical science is the failure, litcrally through centuries, to
utilize the powers of the microscope to promote
the study of morbid anatomy. Shortly after the
Dutch invention of the compound microscope,
whether by the Janssens of Middleburgh or
Drebbel of Alkmaar, it was being used con-
structively in the study of normal animal tissues.
Malpighi's (1628-94) discoveries of the capillaries, the kidney glomeruli, the splenic corpuscles that bear his name, Swammerdam's and
Leeuwenhoek's similar studies of erythrocytes,
spermatozoa, muscle, the crystalline lens, micro-
organisms, as well as the seventeenth-century
productions in botany and zoology by Hooke,
Grew, Athanasius Kircher and others, all these
should have been sufficient to launch a host of
contributions that could easily have advanced
rational medicine by more than a century. But
eighteenth-century theories and systems developed on other lines and, as we have seen,
Morgagni, the Hunters, Bichat and even many of
the clinician-pathologists of the early nineteenth
century owed little or nothing to the microscope. It was not until well in the nineteenth
century that with the aid of the newly invented
achromatic lens the cell was established as the
structural and functional unit of both plant and
animal tissue.

This Cell Theory of living structure, though advanced chiefly by botanists, and a normal rather than a disease concept that is more appropriately taken up elsewhere, is of such fundamental importance to Cellular Pathology that it must be considered here. The cell-like cavities in plant tissues had been known since the seventeenth century (Nehemiah Grew). The mammalian ovum was discovered by von Baer in 1827; and the cell nucleus by Robert Brown in 1831, the year in which *M. J. Schleiden* (1804-81) demonstrated that plants are made up of cells in which the nuclei are important structures. To that versatile genius, *Johannes Müller,* is due much of the stimulus for the new advance. Not only did he make numerous microscopic observations of his own, also achieving the generalization of the correspondence between embryonic and pathologic development; but it was one of his pupils,* *Theodor Schwann* (1810-82), who having seen nucleated cells in animal tissues, was led to the doctrine of the cell structure of animal tissue. Having made a systematic study of all animal tissues, he was able to establish both the similarity of animal and plant tissues and the basic importance of cells in their structure and function (1839). Like Rokitansky, however, he believed that new cells arose from the accumulation of a formation fluid, "the blasteme," giving rise to nucleolus then nucleus and cytoplasm, a concept overthrown by the discovery of mitosis (whence Virchow's *"omnis cellula e cellula"*).

* Henle, Kölliker, duBois Reymond, Helmholtz and Brücke add to the list of Müller's famous pupils, a galaxy only equalled by those of Germany's great physiologist, Karl Ludwig.

New facts about microscopic anatomy accumulated rapidly. Henle within a few years had described various types of epithelium and their function, the muscular coats of arteries and of the bladder, the eponymic loops of the kidney, the structure of hair, the cornea and larynx, as well as many structures in the brain. (As a direct contributor to pathology he was the author of a "Handbuch der rationellen Pathologie" and joint founder of the important *Zeitschrift für rationelle Medizin*.) Nor was the application to pathologic anatomy wanting. By 1843 *Julius Vogel* (1814-80) had brought out his "Icones histologicae pathologicae," divided into two parts that may be likened to general and special pathologic histology, and two years later appeared the "Physiologie pathologique" by *Hermann Lebert* of Breslau.

Thus we see that, as usual, to use Virchow's own words about the cell theory and spontaneous generation, "no development of any kind begins *de novo*." Knowledge of animal cells was accumulating, and yet it is Virchow who is rightly regarded as the apostle of that new doctrine, both for his numerous individual contributions and his masterly generalization of the problem.

Rudolph Ludwig Karl Virchow (1821-1905), the greatest figure in pathology of all time, came under Johannes Müller's influence while a student in Berlin, and thus early saw the possibilities of anatomical study. The year after his graduation he became assistant prosector to *Robert Froriep* (1804-61) at the Charité Hospital; and when Froriep left Berlin for Weimar in 1846, Virchow succeeded him as prosector. In Vir-

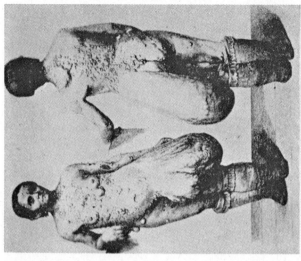

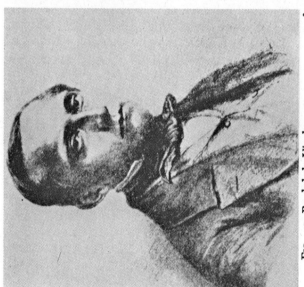

FIG. 13. Rudolph Virchow as a young professor (courtesy of E. R. Long), and the frontispiece of his book on tumors.

chow's twenty-fifth year, 1845, appeared his second paper, one on "Weisses Blut" (leucemia). Though coming out one month later than Bennett's report of a case of suppuration of the blood, Virchow's deserves the greater praise for his correct interpretation that the myriads of leucocytes were not pus corpuscles. It was not long, too, before he distinguished between the spleno-myelogenous and lymphatic forms. The next year his criticism of Rokitansky's *Crases* (the last gasp of the ancient humoral system) in the *Berliner klinische Wochenschrift* so wrecked that system that even Rokitansky himself was forced to abandon it. Virchow's original observations accumulated rapidly; he first published in Froriep's *Notizen*, and in Traube's short-lived *Beiträge zur experimentellen Pathologie*. Its death after 2 volumes led the young Virchow in 1847, together with a gifted young colleague, *Benno Reinhardt* (1820-52), to found the *Archiv für pathologische Anatomie und Physiologie und für klinische Medizin*, which as the familiar *Virchow's Archiv* has continued ever since to occupy a leading position among pathological journals. It is worth noting that, although Virchow and his followers have been wrongly reproached with confining pathology to pure morphology, his journal has always emphasized in its title pathological physiology and the relation of pathology to clinical medicine. Throughout his life Virchow delved in political reform. In the troublous times of 1848, his revolutionary sympathies were too much for the Prussian Government. His removal from Berlin in 1849 was Wurzburg's and probably also Virchow's opportunity. Becoming professor of pathology there he put in seven valuable years before his recall to Berlin, laying the basis for his really epoch-making book, "Die Cellular-pathologie in ihrer Begründung auf physiologische und pathologische Gewebelehre" (1858), which will be considered shortly. The Charité prosectorship having been vacated by the deaths of Reinhardt and *Heinrich Meckel* (1821-56), Johannes Müller secured the creation of the Berlin chair in pathological anatomy, with Virchow as its occupant and director of the new Pathological Institute.

On Schwann's already established cell theory of animal structure, and the doctrine of the continuity of cell life, as represented by the axiom *"Omnis cellula e cellula,"* Virchow rapidly erected the first correctly rational system of disease mechanism that the world had known. This was to make pathology not only the leading medical science for a generation or more, but for all time the basic study of disease by which all advances in ancillary subjects had to be tested and supported. Instead of wholly fanciful systems or of unrelated gross observations or of Rokitansky's tissue changes governed by a controlling "blastema," he firmly established the cell as the all-important unit on which and in which disease processes are active. A "dyscrasia" such as syphilis was correctly regarded as having a local origin in a focus (Herde) from which its noxious matter spread through the body. First combating Cruveilhier's doctrine that phlebitis was the all-important cause of disease, Virchow was led to the elucidation of thrombosis, embolism and pyemia ("Thrombose und Embolie," 1846).

Thrombosis he explained as due to a slowing of the vascular current from compression, dilatation or asthenia and not to inflammation within the veins. Observing a central, puriform softening of the thrombotic mass, he noted that fragments might be detached (which he named emboli), which caused distant damage as soon as they reached vessels of a diameter smaller than their own. This not only led the way to a proper understanding of pyemia (though for the proof of its existence in puerperal fever he was forced to utilize the statistical method of Louis), but also furnished to others the explanation of cancer metastases, which had been regarded as local transformations of tissue through a cancerous secretion.

Virchow's "Cellular Pathologie" represents the short-hand report of twenty lectures given that same year to an assemblage of medical men, as "the time at my disposal was not sufficient to enable me to write out and revise a work like this." Thus was one of the most important books in the history of medicine composed! Written with the double purpose of recording his observations and instructing the medical world in the cellular nature of vital processes as opposed to "the one-sided humoral and neuristical (solidistic) tendencies" transmitted from antiquity, it naturally emphasizes the cellular point of view. A full third of the book is devoted to normal histology. As one would expect with such a pioneer penetration into an unexplored field, mistakes are not infrequent, but they are quite overshadowed by the invaluable concepts and observations that are set forth.

Discussing the *actions* of cells, he first took up inflammation, whose basic importance he early recognized. The cardinal symptoms of Celsus he subordinated to the all-important, *functio laesa,* or damaged function, a dynamic concept that had been announced by Galen but later forgotten. He maintained that an irritated artery in its reaction produced ischemia (see Wharton Jones), and that it was the tissue irritants that increased the bulk of the part whether vessels were present or not. His inaugural dissertation was on inflammation in the avascular cornea. Hyperemia, which he admitted inaugurates the process in all vascular parts, he found localized to the irritated area. Even the inflammatory exudate he explained away as "essentially composed of the material that has been generated in the inflamed part itself." Thus he avoided the classical and Cruveilhian fallacies of the dominance of plethora, but prolonged an error that was only to be rectified by Cohnheim's experiments. Attention concentrated on the single cell and its nutritive state, he developed a whole new field of concepts in relation to its *passive state*: the cell degenerations. The inflamed cell, which had morbidly absorbed excessive fluid, was to him the basic factor in inflammation. An early stage, such as is seen in Bright's disease in the large cloudy kidney epithelium with indistinct nucleus, he designated "cloudy swelling," which gave rise to the term "parenchymatous degeneration." That even the fighter, Virchow, could defer to prevalent opinion is shown by the fact that at first he gave this concept the meaningless term, "parenchymatous exudation," but later changed it to "parenchymatous inflammation." This, the degenerative phase of inflammation, still holds a place in modern, especially German, pathology. Virchow clearly defined fatty degeneration, a necrobiotic process that he found in muscle, arteries, kidney, brain and even liver, the morbid nature of which he correctly distinguished from normal fat tissue and from the physiological fat found in intestinal villi and the liver. The century-old "lardaceous change" (applied even to tumors) he described as amyloid, because like starch it gave a blue color with iodine. He recognized its complex, possible protein nature and that it was conveyed from a distance to be deposited between the tissues.

In the discussion of new formation—a broader concept than neoplasms alone—Virchow emphasized the simple but all-important doctrine of *"continuous development of tissues out of one another,"* as opposed to Rokitansky's blastema or plastic lymph or Schleiden's concept that nuclei first form in a fluid and that membranes later develop about them. He recognized the difference between hypertrophy (an increase in nutrition [size] of existing parts) and hyperplasia (the formation of new elements). Osseous tissue was correctly differentiated from bone as an organ, on the one hand, and from osteoid tissue (uncalcified), on the other. He almost (p. 414 of Cellular Pathologie) recognized the blood-cell-forming function of the red marrow; a discovery reserved for Neumann a decade later (1868). He was familiar with the irregular overgrowth of osteoid tissue and failure to calcify in rickety bones.

In the field of the tumors Virchow always was

deeply interested and to it he made numerous valuable contributions that culminated in his "Die krankhaften Geschwulste" (1863-67). Correct evaluation today of the views that he propounded, however, is made more difficult by his frequent coupling of neoplastic and non-neoplastic new formations. He divided all new formations into *homologous*: those "reproducing the type of the parent soil," such as uterine fibroids; and *heterologous*: those deviating from the recognized type, such as cancer and tubercle. Heterologous he recognized as usually destructive, but —strange mistake for one who so emphasized the unity of the cell—he believed that cells could easily be transformed in nature (metaplasia), and thus derived epithelial carcinomata from connective tissue.

Strange also for one who had solved the problem of embolism and infarction, he was wrong (in his earlier days at least) in his concept of metastasis. The fact that mammary cancer was more frequently followed by secondary cancer of the liver than of the lung seemed to argue against a corpuscular transmission, so that he was unfortunately led to attribute it to certain fluids that "possess the power of producing an infection which disposes different parts to a reproduction of" the parent mass! Thus even genius can be led astray by incorrect though reasonable deductions. He also retarded knowledge of inflammation by rejecting the concept of the migration of leucocytes, he upheld the duality of tuberculosis (though he was well acquainted with its histology), he denied Darwin's theory of evolution and combated the new discoveries in bacteriology and immunology. On the credit side, to quote Garrison: "he also did good work on trichinosis (1859-70), and discovered the sarcinic and aspergillic forms of mycosis in the lungs and bronchial tubes. He also pointed out the true relationship between lupus and tuberculosis, introduced new pathological concepts such as agenesia, heterotopia, ochronosis and first described leontiasis ossea, hematoma of the dura mater, the aortic hypoplasia with contracted heart in chlorotic maidens (1872) and spina bifida occulta (1875). In 1861, he gave the name 'arthritis deformans' to rheumatic gout."

His scientific contributions came in the first fifty years of his life. A multitude of interests—politics (which he reëntered in 1862), anthropology (his hobby), public health, editing and teaching, and the honors that poured upon him were sufficient to account for an existence that remained busy almost to the end without the assumption of any senile let up. But his ·epoch-making contribution to medical progress had been completed before the Franco-Prussian war. W. H. Welch did not hesitate to say that "the establishment by Virchow of the principles of cellular pathology marked the greatest advance which scientific medicine had made since its beginning." Other minds and other better technical methods were required to further the advance of pathology, a branch of science which, after being established as medicine's basic discipline, was soon to hand over the leadership in medical progress to other lines of attack. His pupils who reached distinction are too numerous to mention. Cohnheim, the greatest, figures in the last

chapter of this book; Klebs and Ponfick are associated chiefly with bacteriology; Hoppe-Seyler
and Salkowski with bio-chemistry; some are still
living.

In pathology among the most important was
Friedrich Daniel von Recklinghausen (1833-
1910), who during his thirty odd years' incum-
bency in the Strasbourg chair, made it one of the
leaders of the new school. He is chiefly known for
his description of the eponymic neurofibromatosis
(1881) which had the special merit of outlining
a whole group of fibroid tumors of neural
origin (*cf.* Masson's argentaffin neuromata).
Equally important was his elaboration of his master's study of thrombosis, emboli and infarction
and his clarification of the general subject of bone
pathology (luetic periostitis, osteitis deformans,
osteomalacia, rickets and the carcinomatous stimulation of bone growth). He named and described hemochromatosis, established the lymphoid nature of the green tumor, chloroma, and
traced uterine adenomyoma embryologically. Of
scarcely less importance was *Eduard Rindfleisch*
(1836-1908) whose textbook (1867-69) was
widely used; another was *Johannes Orth* (1847-
1902), who after a long assistantship, succeeded
his teacher at Berlin.

Prominent among the leaders in the new science was *Carl Weigert* (1845-1904), who, taught
by both Virchow and Cohnheim, before he was
thirty had established the nature of the smallpox skin lesions and thus eventually of coagulation necrosis (Cohnheim's term). His technical
discoveries of differential staining (bacteria in
tissues, myelin sheaths, elastic tissue and so on)

permitted noteworthy advances in all these fields; while his generalization that destroyed parenchyma was replaced by an overgrowth of connective tissue has replaced Virchow's concept of parenchymatous and interstitial inflammation, even though we still hear echoes of the latter in such obsolescent terms as chronic interstitial myocarditis or nephritis.

CHAPTER VII

INTEGRATED PATHOLOGY

(STRUCTURAL, FUNCTIONAL, CHEMICAL, EXPERIMENTAL AND CLINICAL METHODS OF APPROACH)

WE HAVE traced the progress of Pathology from the earliest halting observations, through the copious though sporadic collection of Morgagni, the systematized voluminous studies of Rokitansky, and the tissue concepts of Bichat, to the goal of pathologic histology—the cellular pathology of Virchow and his successors. There remains to consider what might be termed a rational or integrated pathology, though "rational" is a term that has been used more than once in such connections with different meanings (*cf.* Henle's "Handbuch der rationellen Pathologie"). Here let us take it to indicate the study of the nature and manifestations of disease by a wise combination of all suitable means available: anatomical, microscopic, functional, bacteriological, chemical, experimental and clinical. Though some such combinations have not been wanting in the past, their planned and persistent coordination may properly be regarded as one of the happy developments of twentieth century medical progress. Whether or not forced upon us by the increasing difficulties in the way of further advances, the combined attack has become more and more frequently the accepted method of approach. Today most worthwhile investigations must be pursued either by group cooperation or by the superman who is a sufficient master in various branches to utilize any combination of methods that the problem requires.

One of these methods, experimental pathology, remains to be considered. Pathological experiments have been made sporadically by the unusual individual since classical times. *Galen's* production of hemiplegia and of different paralyses by various sections of the spinal cord and of aphonia by cutting the recurrent laryngeal nerve come first to mind, while study of the effect of poisons on slaves or animals was a practical necessity in all ages. Other experiments doubtless were performed and recorded, but in general the classical Greeks depended mostly on theory and observation and the Arabs and scholars of the Middle Ages on tradition. In the freer air of the Renaissance experiments began to be designed to test new thoughts and some of these were in the domain of pathology. *Giuseppe Zambeccari* in 1680 described the successful removal of dog's spleens (of course, without any thought of producing blood changes thereby), and he also removed various other organs. ("Esperimenti intorno le diverse viscere togliate a diversi animali viventi" quoted by Morgagni). *Richard Lower* (1631-91) tested the effect of transfusing blood from one animal to another,* and demonstrated the nature of the mechanical form of edema by simply tying off the vein to a part. He even ligated the vena cava in some experiments. *Regnier de Graaf* (1641-73) studied

---

* Pepys' entertaining account of this performance is one of many indications of the hold that budding scientific investigation had on the seventeenth century lay mind.

the effects of parotid and pancreatic fistulae, while *J. C. Brunner* (1653-1727) removed the spleen and pancreas of dogs and nearly anticipated the discovery of the cause of diabetes (1683) by over two centuries. Deductions, to be sure, were often faulty, as in *Willis'* incorrect ascription of various cerebral functions after experimental damage to the cerebellum.

Animal experimentation on a large scale was introduced by the versatile *Haller*, who among his innumerable physiological experiments first studied the fate of septic material injected into the body, and also the results of interfering with the muscular transmission of the cardiac impulse. Nevertheless, his small "Opuscula pathologica" (1768) contains but eighty short observations that are far from the most important of his countless scientific papers. The first of its four plates shows a fine fusiform aneurysm of the aortic arch, the earliest I have found; the third depicts both a corpus luteum and a very early fetus. Contemporary with Haller, *Robert Whytt* (1714-66) was exploring the pathologic physiology of the nervous system, through his studies of spinal shock and the abolition of the (Whytt's) pupillary reflex to light (1768) by destruction of the anterior corpa quadrigemina. Similarly the dog experiments (1769) of *Nicholas Saucerotte* (1714-1814) explained the contralateral paralysis following cerebral injury a century before the development of technical methods permitted its microscopic demonstration. This observing surgeon also noted the comparative silence of anterior cerebral injuries, "described the neighborhood symptoms in cerebral compression by blood clots, the periodic coma and gigantism in acromegaly (1772) and noted the opisthotonos, hyperesthesia and nystagmus in cerebellar lesions." (Garrison.)

Pieter Camper (1722-89) better known for his anatomical studies and illustrations, was also a surgeon of note. The first to conduct a surgical polyclinic, he exemplified the investigating spirit by cutting the symphysis in animals with prompt healing, to the frustration of the opponents of symphysiotomy.

These are obviously but a few isolated examples of the experimental study of pathology before Hunter, but their importance to us lies partly in the fact that they were but sporadic and isolated.

Admittedly the greatest of experimental biologists was that eccentric British genius, *John Hunter* (1728-93). A life-long, insatiable curiosity directed his experiments into the most varied fields and on all sorts of animals, including himself. In fact his tragic death from angina pectoris was probably the result of his self-inoculation with material from a person suffering from venereal disease. This experiment proved a good example of the truth of the Hippocratic dictum that experience is difficult. Unfortunately choosing a subject that had both gonorrhea and syphilis, he was led to the false conclusion of the identity of the two diseases, a conclusion that retarded knowledge of venereal disease by a half century, until corrected by *Philippe Ricord* (1799-1899), a great French venereologist, born in Baltimore, "the Voltaire of pelvic literature"

(O. W. Holmes), permanently established their separate natures (1838).

Shortly after coming to London from their home in Lanarkshire (1748) to study and assist his brother in dissecting and to study surgery with Cheselden and Pott, John began his original investigations in the most varied fields. For him Terence's aphorism might be paraphrased: "Nothing biological do I regard as alien to me." With the surgical experience gained in the expedition to Belle Isle (1761), he amassed a considerable surgical practice, which, pursued in conjunction with his ardent investigations, carried surgery to a leading position in the British medical sky. As Garrison phrases it, he "found surgery a mechanical art and left it an experimental science." Fortunately ignorant of the confusing medical theories and systems that flooded the eighteenth century, and taught chiefly in the school of practical experience, Hunter devised experiments that were simple but led to adequate, sometimes important answers. His attitude is summed up in his well-known advice to Jenner: "But why think, why not try the experiment?" And yet it is no disparagement to agree that his exalted position in British biology is due more to his constant insistence on experimentation than to any new approach to the study of biology or to the actual discoveries that he accomplished.

Among his chief achievements were the studies on the formation of pus and the function of the lymphocytes, on the depression of function (digestion) during hibernation, on the collateral circulation in deer's antlers (which led to an

improved method of ligating aneurysms) and
successful grafting of cock's spurs on their combs.
His chief publications were on the "Natural
History of the Human Teeth" (1771) ; "Venereal
Disease" (1786) ; "Certain Parts of the Animal
Oeconomy" (1786) and, posthumously published, "The Blood, Inflammation and Gunshot
Wounds" (1794). The influence of Hunter's
ideas continues to be felt in England where he
is justly regarded as one of their very greatest
medical figures. His experimental method, however, failed to produce any noteworthy followers
in his own country.

Gradually the idea came to be accepted that
disease processes as well as normal function were
subject to experimental approach. If any one
source can be selected as the origin of the new
tendency, it is the French school begun by
François Magendie (1783-1855) of Bordeaux.
Regarding medicine as a science in the making,
he made experiments and "picked up his scraps"
of observations in the most varied fields. Studies
on the flow of the gastric juice, the mechanism of
swallowing, the absorbent qualities of the blood
vessels, the function of the anterior and posterior
nerve roots and the importance of nitrogenous
foods were augmented in the field of functional
pathology by studies on the effect of damage to
or excision of the cerebellum (1825), of lesions
of the optic thalamus, of injecting putrid matter
into the veins (with Gaspard), and especially
the demonstration of the fatal effects of a second
injection of egg albumen into rabbits (1839),
the phenomenon we now know as anaphylaxis.

Not the least of his achievements was the stim-

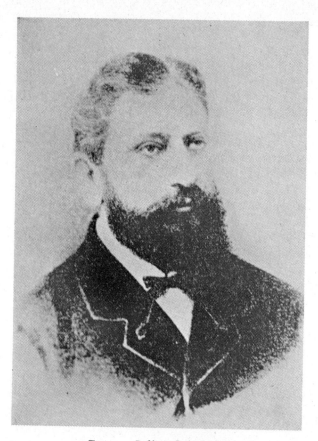

Fig. 14. Julius Cohnheim.
(From a charcoal sketch.)

ulation of his far greater pupil, *Claude Bernard* (1813-78), whose "Introduction à l'étude de la médecine expérimentale," though written by a professional physiologist, inaugurated a new era in pathology—the systematic experimental study of disease phenomena in the living. As valuable today as under the far different conditions in which it was written, this book not only contains an unexcelled statement of the philosophy of experimental reasoning but outlines the principles of an animal experimentation designed to further all branches of medical science. Bernard's concept of the *"milieu internale"* is only today becoming properly recognized as a basic principle in the interrelationship of the viscera, especially the endocrine organs, and their disorders. His discovery of the glycogenic function of the liver (1849) (an internal secretion, in his own words) was basic for a modern concept of diabetes, while his "piqure" of the fourth ventricle (1850) produced glycosuria in another startling fashion. His demonstration of the importance of pancreatic digestion (1849-56) has obvious pathologic applications; while the demonstration of the vasomotor mechanism (1851-53) and the vasoconstrictor and dilator nerves opened further vistas of medical advance. He also showed that carbon-monoxide poisoning is due to the replacement of the oxygen in the erythrocyte. Among his pupils were his successor Paul Bert, Brown-Séquard, Russell Chittenden and Willy Kühne.

Through Kühne his influence can be traced to the latter's pupil, *Julius Cohnheim* (1839-84), unquestionably the master experimental pathologist of the modern era. Virchow's most distinguished pupil, Cohnheim throughout a short but active life emphasized and illuminated the functional and experimental study of disease, both while assistant to Virchow at Berlin and while occupying the chairs of Kiel (1868-72), Breslau (1872-78), and Leipzig (1878-84). His magnificent "Lectures on General Pathology" (1877) (available in English in the New Sydenham Society translation) remains a modern book, in a way that is quite lacking in Virchow's "Cellular Pathology" or Rokitansky's "Handbuch." "A bright and jovial student, full of drollery" (Immermann), at Wurzburg, Greifswald and Berlin, Cohnheim prepared himself well for his life's work. Long hours with the microscope, under the guidance of Kölliker in normal and of Virchow in morbid histology, gave him the necessary structural foundation for his experimental work. His Inaugural Dissertation, "De pyogenesi in tunicis serosis," inaugurated one of his chief efforts. In this great battlefield—the nature of inflammation—he was able to support his master's contribution that the pus-corpuscle and the leucocyte were identical. However, with the ingenious use of dyes he correctly derived the leucocyte from the blood, Virchow believing that it was a local tissue cell. "That pus is formed in the capillary vessels by a process analogous to secretion was first suggested by Dr. Simpson of St. Andrews, in the year 1722." (Carswell). With his well-known frog mesentery experiment, Cohnheim was next able actually to see the leucocyte escaping from the vessel wall, together with the attendant phenomena of widening of the lumen, slowing of the current and diapedesis of erythrocytes—a forgotten observation of Addison (1849) and Waller. "Ohne Gefässe keine Entzundung," said Cohnheim, thus undermining his master, Virchow's, tenets in favor of the earlier discarded views. It was not, however, until Metchnikoff's discovery (1884) of the macrophage and microphage (the pus cell from the blood) and the true explanation of inflammatory phenomena in avascular tissues that a proper combination of vascular and tissue phases of inflammation could be made. In the stimulating atmosphere of the Charité laboratories, Cohnheim continued his master's studies on emboli and venous stasis and introduced valuable improvements in technique, such as frozen microscopic sections, staining muscle nerve endings with silver salts, and corneal nerve endings with gold. At Breslau, the chance observation of a case of congenital kidney sarcoma suggested to him the theory that cancer was due to misplaced embryonal rests. At Breslau also were performed with Salomonsen his successful inoculations of tuberculous material into the rabbit's eye, where the transparent, closed chamber allowed observation of the development of the tubercle.

As with Carl Ludwig, his intellect also was productive through his pupils, Lassar, Heidenhain, Litten, Ehrlich, Neisser, Weigert, and, of especial interest to Americans, *William Welch* (1850-1934), who while studying under Cohnheim at Breslau completed his study of acute edema of the lungs. Other investigations by the clear sighted Welch followed in this country (discovery of *B. aerogenes capsulatus* and exploration of its pathologic effects, further advances in

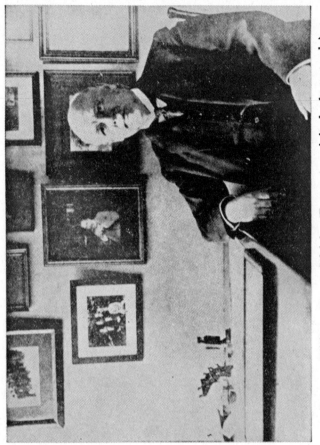

FIG. 15. William Henry Welch. (From an original photograph.)

the field of embolism and thrombosis, lesions of diptheria toxin and so on). But vastly more important to the progress of American medicine was the dynamic concept that Welch brought to a profession over-impressed with the importance of pathologic anatomy and his wise guidance not only of his department at Johns Hopkins but of the medical profession of the whole country throughout a long life, influential to the very last.

In the half century following Cohnheim's death, the volume of experimental work permitted by the numerous well-equipped pathologic institutes, together with the better correlation of clinical and pathologic observation by pathologically trained minds, has produced many notable discoveries as well as a rapid, sound exploitation of the new observations. In the field of the *glands of internal secretion* has this been especially marked. Diabetes, for instance, known but not understood for centuries, was produced experimentally by the clinicians, *von Mering* and *Minkowski*, by removing the dog's pancreas (1889); Minkowski having already studied the acidotic urine of diabetes (1884), and the former having produced glycosuria with phlorhizin (1886). *Opie's* and *McCallum's* pathologic histological studies connected the pancreas with human diabetes, and its nature was further elucidated by the chemical studies of *Naunyn* (who introduced the term "acidosis"), *Magnus-Levy* and others. But it was not until 1921 that the experiments of *Banting* and *Best* isolated insulin from the pancreas. The part that other endocrine organs play in the diabetic process is now being actively investigated. Similarly several specialties contributed to the study of exophthalmic goiter and myxedema: known clinically since the first and third quarters of the nineteenth century, respectively, their essential connection with dysfunction of the thyroid gland was indicated (1859-84) in the dog experiments of *Moritz Schiff* (1823-96) (removal of the thyroid with subsequent thyroid grafts or administration of thyroid extract). In the hands of *Theodor Kocher*, the new "physiological surgery" showed that in man thyroidectomy could both relieve the overproduction symptoms of exophthalmic goiter and produce a myxedematous state (cachexia strumipriva). Experimental surgery (*Sir Victor Horsley*) showed that this cachexia, myxedema and cretinism were all due to lack of thyroid secretion. The chemical nature of the active agent was established by *Baumann's* (1896) discovery of iodothyrin and *E. C. Kendall's* (1914) isolation of the actual crystalline substance, thyroxin.

The superficially insignificant parathyroids were longer in acquiring evaluation. Practically unrecognized till 1880 (Sandström), their necessity for life was first shown by *Gley* in 1891 in connection with experimental thyroidectomy. Their relation to tetany evolved from the surgeon *von Eiselsberg's* experimental thyroidectomies published the next year, and this avenue later linked them with calcium metabolism (*MacCallum and Voigtlin*, 1908). Biochemistry contributed discovery of the active principle—parathormone (*Collip*, 1926); the happy combination of clinical medicine and surgery with biochemistry and pathologic anatomy being again emphasized when osteitis fibrosa cystica was shown to be due to excessive parathyroid secretion that could be relieved by removal of a parathyroid tumor or hyperplastic gland (*Mandl, Barr, Albright, et al.*).

Of equal interest is the story of pituitary pathology. Though isolated lesions had been observed for centuries (at least as far back as Bonetus' "Sepulchretum"), the pituitary was not correlated with clinical disease until *Mohr* described obesity with pituitary tumor (1840). *Marie* found pituitary tumors in acromegaly (1886) and the skeletons of giants were found to have enlarged pituitary fossae. In 1901, *Fröhlich* described the adiposo-genital dystrophy of pituitary origin; in 1914, *Simmonds* the pituitary type of dwarfism; and in 1929, *Harvey Cushing* outlined the syndrome that is associated with tumor of the basophilic cells of the anterior lobe. In the meantime, experimental pathology has not only reproduced many of these clinical conditions, but has shown such important relationships to other glands of internal secretion, that the pituitary has been aptly termed "the conductor of the endocrine orchestra."

Integrated pathology has played a prominent part in the recent advances in the field of the *Vitamins*. Pellagra, rickets and scurvy had been known, to be sure, for centuries, but it was not until the combined contributions of the clinicians, *Eijkmann* and *Hess*, the biochemists, *Hopkins* and *McCollum*, the pathologists, *Goldberger* and *Wolbach*, and others too numerous to mention, that we have been able to correlate such diseases with lack of this or that vitamin, to understand their nature and often to make headway in overcoming them. It is in these two groups, the endocrine diseases and the avitaminoses, that recent progress has been most active and the advantage of correlated study has been most conclusively demonstrated. Limitations of space prevent consideration of the achievements of integrated pathology in other fields, such as acidosis, disordered mechanisms of metabolism, of osmosis and of the nicely balanced physico-chemical equilibria of the blood; but it is obvious that it is destined to achieve further triumphs in rapid succession.

CHAPTER VIII

SPECIAL CONCEPTS: INFLAMMATION, CANCER

O F THE major processes that constitute what we now understand as General Pathology, two, namely inflammation and cancer, are so much the most important, both from the point of view of their prevalence in disease as well as their long and varied history, that it is desirable to review briefly the views that have been held regarding them.

INFLAMMATION

The group of changes which we now include under the concept Inflammation has been a focus of medical interest since the earliest times; in fact, only the bare essentials can be indicated here, scarcely enough to serve as a guide to one wishing to survey the topic adequately. Indeed so complex had the subject become a century ago that Andral and later Thoma recommended that the whole concept be abandoned.

Even the earliest Egyptian papyri recognized pus as related to the demon of disease and they described abscesses and ulcers. As an easily visible disease condition of the external parts, its manifold manifestations have been well depicted ever since the time of the Hippocratic writers. These keen observers also made the fundamental advance of regarding the patient, not the disease, as the unit, so that his resistance to disease became a more important consideration than the demon or charm. The true nature of disease, however, almost necessarily remained obscure till in the nineteenth century the importance of pathological histology and the rôle played by bacteria and biochemistry became appreciated. During the long sway of the classical humoral pathology (q.v. Chapter 1), inflammation was regarded as the result of the body's effort to return to health by coction of fluids and tissues, pus thus representing blood or other humors heated to the point of putrefaction. The warmth (hence "phlegmon") of the inflamed part, according to the Hippocratic school, was due to the heaping up of the natural warmth that the heart emits, thus producing an increased flow of the humors. But they had no special name for inflammation, "erysipelas" emphasizing the redness and "edema" the swelling. "Apostasis" or "apostema," terms used in almost a hundred places in the Hippocratic Corpus, indicated a deposition of harmful material, beneficial (like fever) when it localized the damage, but sometimes harmful if widespread, as in pyemia. "In most the deposit ends in suppuration" (3 Bk. "Epid.") ; and this also was regarded as desirable, as it damaged the neighboring tissues less and did not recur. Even in fresh wounds, a good and laudable pus was welcomed. Such theories can often be argued into seeming not far wide of the mark in the light of modern knowledge; but this is always more or less due to the unconsciously injected modern point of view. One has only to consider the practical applications usually made of the old theories to see how far removed they were from true concepts.

To Erasistratus, whose entire pathology was built around the concept Plethora, inflammation was due to the blood entering the air-containing arteries from the veins where it became stagnant and compressed by the air from the heart. The swelling came from overloading of the blood vessels of the affected part—one of the manifestations of inflammation, to be sure, but not its cause. Purely fantastical was the application of the *strictum et laxum* theory of Asclepiades and Themison, where imaginary pores were stopped up by equally imaginary atoms.

To Celsus, as has already been noted, we owe the now threadbare cardinal signs of inflammation, with which every medical student is familiar: "Notae vero inflammationis sunt quattuor rubor et tumor cum calore et dolore," which with the "Functio laesa" added by Galen constitute an excellent summary of the chief gross changes. Like Hippocrates, Celsus believed inflammation of wounds to be due to the degeneration of blood into pus.

Galen, the first to write extensively on inflammation ("Ad glauconem de med. meth.," Bk. 2), maintained that stagnation of any of the "humors" might lead to inflammation, with further progression to serous exudate ($\iota\chi\omega\rho$), suppuration and necrosis or gangrene. He distinguished four varieties: Phlegmon (from blood); erysipelas (from yellow bile); edema, cold swellings (from coagulated phlegm) and cancer (from black bile). He made the significant advance that the same result (inflammation) could result from various injuries: wounds, bruises, fractures, ulcers or even when congested veins pour blood into spongy tissue. Lending his authority, however, to the humoral view that "coction" was necessary for the expulsion of bad humors and hence for the healing of inflamed wounds (i.e., suppuration), he gave support to the pernicious doctrine of "laudable pus," a dogma that was maintained till the nineteenth century. De Mondeville and others in the thirteenth century, to be sure, insisted on cleanliness and opposed the healing of wounds by producing suppurations (setons); but his principles were soon forgotten and fifty years later his great successor, Guy de Chauliac, was a conventional believer in laudable pus.

Though descriptions of inflammatory diseases continued with increasing precision, especially in the seventeenth and eighteenth centuries, the pathological concept of inflammation failed to improve. Even the combative Paracelsus followed the concept of apostema, inflammation being a minor variety, due to imbalance of salt sulphur and mercury, instead of the four humors. Sydenham, the English Hippocrates, to be sure, recognized fever as a purifying process, designed to free the blood from the disease, a foreign invader; but his really important contribution was the accurate recognition of morbid states by exact observation of signs and symptoms in the true Hippocratic spirit. The fantastic animistic and tonus theories of Brown and Hoffmann, which exerted great influence for many decades, were but little if at all superior to Erasistratus' plethora or Asclepiades' *"strictum et laxum."* But the idea of contagion was gradually gaining ground and with the basic contributions of Harvey's demonstration of the circulation of the blood and Malpighi's discovery of the capillaries, light was bound to follow.

Considerable differences of opinion existed as to the part played by the tissues and the vessels. The eclectic Boerhaave was aware of the importance of both, so that his teaching has been called a forerunner of cellular pathology, even though his emphasis was on the changed state of the vessels. He stated that all tissues were full of vessels of all sizes, and believed that inflammation arose not only from a changed state of the sanguineous humor but from an excess of blood in the inflamed part due to increased hydrostatic pressure and to the friction of the red arterial blood in the smallest canals. Thus some of the blood was driven faster by the fever that was present, while elsewhere the vessels were filled to such a point that the circulation stopped. To him then inflammation arose from a circulatory disturbance and especially a stasis, in a sense prophetic of Cohnheim's demonstration more than a century later.

Haller's doctrine of irritability was applied to inflammation by his colleague, *J. van Gorter* (1689-1762), who in the first part of his "Compendium medicinae," recognized that the most varied kinds of irritants (of external and internal origin) could *drive* the blood into small vessels and lymphatics and thus cause inflammation.

John Hunter, a pioneer in so many directions, made shrewd deductions from his gross observations in this field ("Treatise on the Blood, Inflammation and Gunshot Wounds") (published posthumously in 1794), though he sometimes lost his way in the treacherous marshes of teleology. Inflammation, being necessarily to him a defensive mechanism whose purpose it was to restore normal function, fell locally into three groups: the adhesive, which prevented the spread of the process; the suppurative, which was designed to rid the blood of harmful material by a process resembling secretion; and ulceration for the removal of dead matter, and often death of the part. Also he recognized that any injury might cause inflammation and that the redness and heat were due to the increased amount of blood flowing through the blood vessels. The coagulable lymph (fibrin), useful in limiting the inflammation, he recognized as coming from the blood, as did pus (though not preexistant there), by a gland-like activity of the vessels. He knew that pus contained corpuscles and that the sedimentation rate of blood was increased in fever. He produced and studied inflammation experimentally. For him the increased blood supply hastened repair. To show that more blood would stimulate growth, he transplanted the spurs of cocks into their combs. (Cheatle, however, has shown that they would grow as fast if transplanted into avascular tissues.)

The important French school took a different stand, namely, that inflammation was itself the disease, and they treated it on this basis. Broussais regarded it as a local fever but believed that the local activity of the vessels was itself faulty. *Gendrin* also wrote extensively on the subject (1826), using the microscope and the classic experimental material: frog mesentery and bat's wing, but failed to appreciate the defensive nature of its reaction. Cruveilhier's concept that abnormal secretions from the blood vessels were responsible for all structural changes fitted inflammation better than it did most lesions. He emphasized the great frequency with which living tissue becomes inflamed and regarded inflammation as due to secretions from the all-powerful capillaries, which had become distended and stagnant. The nature of the inflammation depended on whether the capillaries secreted lymph, pus, caseous material and so on, reminiscent of Hunter's adhesive and suppurative types. Regarding the capillaries as part of the venous system, he allowed that phlebitis one way or another dominated pathology. Though he recognized adhesive and suppurative phlebitis, yet he failed to comprehend such apt illustrations of his concept as embolism and pyemia, which had to await the master touch of Virchow for elucidation. The influence of his views on the immutability of the tissues was a definite retardation of this phase of the subject. His splendid atlas ("L'anatomie pathologique du corps humain," 1829-42), on the other hand, was a landmark in the history of pathologic illustration and played an important part in familiarizing the medical world with pathologic anatomy.

Horner's "Treatise on Pathologic Anatomy" (1829), the first to be published on the subject in this country, illustrates the prevalent ideas on inflammation in the days immediately preceding pathologic histology. The manifestations of phlegmasia (acute inflammation) were still based on Celsus' cardinal signs. In a rapid termination by *"delitescence"* the blood was regarded

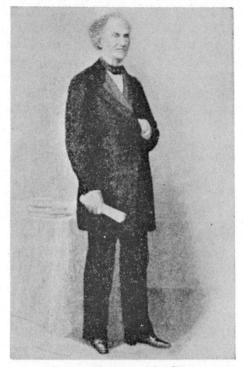

FIG. 16. Samuel Gross, a leading surgeon
who wrote the second American textbook
of Pathology and founded the Philadelphia Pathological Society. (From an original engraving.)

as merely distending the vessels; in the slower termination by "*resolution*," the red blood cells had either ruptured into or percolated into the surrounding tissues. If removal was not accomplished, "the parts take on a secretory action, and discharge pus" (*suppuration*). If in a surface inflammation suppuration is not established, the eroded surface terminates in *ulceration*. If "the afflux of blood to the part ceases . . . but the tumefaction continues to augment by a deposit of the white portions of the blood," termination is by *induration* or *scirrhus* ("in the highly vascular tissues . . . red induration or hepatization"). If "the part affected is absolutely killed," it is called gangrene.

Ten years later, S. D. Gross' "Elements of Pathologic Anatomy" described with detailed lucidity the effusion of serum "which occurs in almost every inflammation." Describing such subdivisions of edema as anasarca, dropsy, hydrocephalus, hydrarthrosis, Gross utilized Marcet's chemical studies of the composition of edematous fluid, properly to derive it from the blood serum. He also recognized certain exceptions to its inflammatory origin. With his naturally close correlation of pathology to surgical affections, he gave good descriptions of the granulation process, "one of the grand operations employed by nature for the cure of wounds," and of cicatrization. As this work was published the same year as Schwann's promulgation of the cell theory of animal tissue, it naturally included no cellular details. Yet both it and Horner's book are good illustrations of a phenomenon frequently to be found in medical history; namely, that without the intervening occurrence of any one important discovery, there is a gradual orientation toward what later becomes established as the correct concept.

Beginnings of microscopic observation of the small vessels in inflammation had been made by Cowper, Haller, Spallanzani and Kaltenbrunner. There was considerable difference of opinion as to the cause and nature of the circulatory disturbances. That the hyperemia was due to an increased distention of the small vessels and not as at first believed to passage of blood into vessels not normally containing blood or the exit of blood into the tissues, was now decided by direct observation. *Vacca* (1765) seems to have been the first to emphasize the importance of local weakness of the vessels that favored the long-recognized stagnation theory.

An important concept was introduced by *Henle's* view that the vessel distention in inflammatory hyperemia was due to a changed innervation of the vessel wall through an irritation of the centripetal nerve. If the centripetal nerve was paralyzed, the effect of the inflammatory stimulus was diminished and following a temporary narrowing of the vessels the distention might go on to complete stoppage of the circulation by vessel paralysis. Only in recent times has the possibility of true inflammation without nervous influence been amply demonstrated. It was also recognized that after the vessel changes, there came a piling up of the well-known white elements of the blood in the surrounding tissues. From this fecund doctrine there was a surprising rebellion led by Goodsir, Redfern and no less a person than Virchow, who wished to ascribe inflammatory phenomena to disturbance of nutrition (parenchymatous inflammation) rather than to circulatory changes. Thus arose Virchow's teaching of the inflamed cell (i.e., cloudy swelling) in parenchymatous inflammation. This was supported by the observed fact that inflammation may also appear in parts that have no vessels: as for instance in the increase of epithelium and pus cells in inflammation of the cornea and the changes in the intima of the aorta, neither of which contains vessels. Yet about 1870, Burdon Sanderson gave a definition of inflammation based on John Hunter's views that is practically the one in general use today: he stated that inflammation is the succession of changes occurring in a part as the result of an injury, provided that the injury be not so excessive as to destroy the vitality of the part. Compare this with Menkin's definition of 1935 as "the complex vascular, lymphatic and general tissue response to the presence of an irritant."

The rediscovery by Cohnheim of the exudation of the leucocytes from the blood vessels in inflammation reestablished on a permanent basis the preeminent rôle played by the blood vessels and their contents, though it put too far in the background the active share of the tissue cells in the inflammatory process. The exudation process had been appreciated by William Addison in 1842 ("Blood Corpuscles, Inflammation and the Origin and Mode of Tubercles in the Lungs"), who recognized "pus corpuscles as altered colorless blood corpuscles," rather than as previously believed, accumulations of granules. The importance of the blood vessels was not firmly established, however, until Cohnheim's classical experiments on the frog's cornea and mesentery gave direct microscopic evidence, not only of the changes occurring in the blood vessels, but of the migration of leucocytes from the blood vessels into the tissues, even though relatively distant (1867-73) (see preceding chapter). Further differentiation of cells, chiefly through the technical staining discoveries of Ehrlich, showed, as every medical student now knows, that cells of various kinds, some arising in the inflamed area and some coming from the blood stream, take part in the inflammatory process, both by direct phagocytosis (Metchnikoff's macrophage and microphage), by liberation of enzymes and by other physico-chemical processes. A satisfactory middle-of-the-road explanation was thus reached between the extremes of circulatory and cellular theories. But the importance of the unsolved problems of this fundamental process continues to impress pathologists; in the year in which I write, inflammation is announced as the chief topic of our national society's program. Developments too recent to consider historically are the rôle of local and general allergy, the rôle of the lymphatics and of mechanical fixation of an irritant in the tissues (Menkin) and the nature of the stimulant to the circulatory response (Lewis' "H substance"). Thus while the etiology and pathologic anatomy of inflammation may be fairly well understood, about its pathogenesis and the far-reaching consequences of its functional effects on the organism there is still much to be learned.

CANCER

Cancer, which with inflammation forms the most important of pathological concepts, has an equally long and varied history, which is even more complicated by a multiplicity of terms used in different senses. Superficial tumors or neoplasms must, of course, have been recognized from the earliest times; but, as the Latin name "tumor" implies, many swellings other than neoplasms were included, even until the more precise days of the nineteenth century. "Praeter naturam," "phymata," "carcinoma," "sarcoma," and so on, all terms in use since classical times, require a specialist's knowledge to give them proper evaluation through the centuries.

Cancer is mentioned in the Ebers Papyrus where, as in the Indian Ramayana, the ulcerating forms were treated with a paste containing arsenic known as "Egyptian" ointment, a remedy that continued popular till the seventeenth century. There is a clear description of a lipoma, treated "with the knife." One of the earliest references to cancer in Assyria is a cuneiform inscription of about 800 B.C. concerning cancer of the breast under the name "machsu." A frequently quoted instance of cancer of the breast was recorded by Democedes (520 B.C.) in the cure of Atossa, the daughter of Darius; as a $\varphi\hat{v}\mu\alpha$, however, this may have been some other form of chronic swelling.

Votive offerings of cancer of the breast and other organs were to be found in pre-Hippocratic temples, as they are in many Roman Catholic churches today. The Hippocratic School has given us many good descriptions of neoplasms (skin, breast, stomach, uterus, rectum, and so on) and an attempt at classification which still persists. From them comes "καρκίνωμα" a progressive malignant tumor, as opposed to "καρκίνος": any ulcer that did not heal normally, terms suggested by the finger-like projections resembling the legs of a crab, though Setinus also suggests its crab-like adherence to the tissues. The word "κίρρος" had the same significance as is attached to it to-day, of a hard perhaps nodular growth. They recognized that "occult" (probably deepseated, non-ulcerating) cancers did better without such treatment as was then available.

Celsus wrote of carcinoma as an immovable irregular tumor, that should be treated with medicines or cautery or excision, but recognized that often treatment was useless. He classified malignant disease as: first (and least) "cacoethes," then carcinoma without ulceration and finally the ulcerating or most malignant form. He is said to have "stressed the involvement of the axillary glands in mammary carcinoma" and left a good picture of carcinoma of the skin. *Leonides of Alexandria* (*ca.* 180 A.D.), known only through the references in Aetius—was said to be the first to recognize nipple retraction in mammary cancer, which he treated vigorously.

From Galen, however, came the classification which persisted for over a thousand years: As opposed to the *"tumores secundam naturam"* (physiological swellings such as the gravid uterus) and *"tumores supra naturam"* (mostly proliferative inflammations, hyperplasias, monstrosities), were *"tumores praeter naturam"* or neoplasms, as we term them today, though cysts and various inflammatory swellings were also included. Galen held that such tumors were due to an excess of black bile, which solidified in certain elective sites, such as the lips, tongue and breast. They were to be got rid of with purgatives that dissolved the black bile, but if this failed, to be cut out, being careful to get all the roots ("De meth. med.," XIII). He, however, was not cognizant of internal forms of cancer, which were discovered sometime between 200 and 600 A.D. (Alexander of Tralles), nor with metastases or extension by the lymphatics. He employed the term "sarcoma" (σάρξ, flesh) for any fleshy-like superficial swelling.

In the Byzantine period cancer received considerable attention. Aetius (502-575), though compiling largely from Archigenes and Leonidas, gave good descriptions of the signs and symptoms of extensive cancer of the breast (retraction of the nipple) and of the uterus (cervical discharge, and so on), always distinguishing in description and treatment between the ulcerating and non-ulcerating forms. Paul of Aegina (625-690) devoted a section to cancer (Bk. IV, Sect. 26), which he says occurs in every part of the body. He was a complete atrabilist in theory.

The Arabians, too, adhered to the atrabilic theory of cancer but were divided as to forms of treatment. As has frequently been noted, however, Avenzoar gave a clear-cut description of cancer of the stomach (*verruca ventriculi*) and recognized cancer of the esophagus (pain and difficult swallowing, finally complete obstruction), which he treated with silver sounds and nutrient enemas.

Through the Middle Ages, Galen's theory of cancer held sway. Thus Henri de Mondeville excised lymph nodes in cancer, but thought that cancer settled there because the black bile entered spongy tissue more easily than solid. His contemporary, Lanfranc, favored radical incision. Saliceto recognized that surgical treatment often made the cancer worse than before and Guy de Chauliac practiced excision in the early stages and cautery in the fungating types, as well as using caustic pastes. Both were thorough Galenists, however, in their concepts of pathogenesis.

Benivieni's book, previously referred to, includes one obvious example (Case 36) of carcinoma of the pylorus, *stomachum abcalluisse*, where at autopsy an obstructive mass in the stomach was found to be the cause of the persistent vomiting and emaciation that had been found. Paré showed a definite acquaintance with internal forms of cancer and knew of the liability of axillary nodes to be involved in mammary carcinoma. So did Fabricius Hildanus, who is said to have been the first to remove these nodes in mammary cancer. Severinus, the first surgical pathologist, distinguished between benign (struma) and malignant breast tumors. Nevertheless, understanding of the nature of malignant disease did not progress: Fernel called almost any superficial growth that was nodular a sarcoma, and obvious gastric cancer was designated abscess. Tulp, who gave the first good description of cancer of the bladder and described

cancer of the esophagus with stricture, hydatidiform mole and sarcoma of the femur (with re-
currence after sixteen years), regarded cancer
of the breast as contagious. Paracelsus' revolt
from Galen led him to discard the atrabiliary
origin of cancer, only to substitute an equally
fanciful concentration of various mineral salts
of the body.

In Bonetus' great collection, 48 folio pages
are given to tumors *"praeter naturam"*; but as
usual many other conditions than neoplasms are
included. Even Morgagni, who described a number of tumors in various chapters of "De sedibus," including cancers of the esophagus, stomach, rectum, pancreas, adrenal and probably the
prostate, apparently had no conception of tumor
metastasis. The first really good pathological description of cancer of the rectum had been in
Donato's "De medicina" (1586).

During the seventeenth century, the importance to cancer of the newly discovered lymphatics was gradually becoming recognized. The
coagulability of the lymph suggested that cancer might arise in this way; and the French
surgeons, J. L. Petit, Antoine Louis, and especially H. F. le Dran (1685-1770) emphasized in
support of this view the spread of cancer via
the lymphatics, the enlargement of the regional
lymph nodes, and the marked tendency to recur.
Astruc, still from the Galenic point of view, believed that scirrhus came from the lymph, and
that cancer was a product of the lymph through
thickening of the humors. He distinguished cancer from cysts, which he regarded as dilated
lymphatics, and disproved the essential acridity

of the humors in malignancy by comparing chemical analyses of ashed cancer and beef steak. Occupational cancer (chimney sweep's) was first described by Percival Pott (1775).

Bernard Peyrilhe (1735-1804), in his prize-winning academic dissertation (1776), was the first to bring out the relation of scirrhus to cancer. He also recognized the rôle of the lymphatics in the spread of the infection, the secondary infection of ulcerated tumors and was the first to attempt the experimental study of cancer (by injecting cancerous tissue in a dog).

John Hunter believed that every "neoplasia" was started by an effusion from the blood vessels of plastic lymph which was capable of self organization ("Treatise on the Blood," 1794). This was a not unreasonable belief before the days of the cell theory, but it is strange that it should have persisted both in Schwann's cytoblastema and Rokitansky's blastema. Comparing neoplasia to the growth of the chick, Hunter regarded it as a kind of parasite, which, like the embryo, next came to be considered as having its own independently formed vascular system.

The parasite idea was carried so far that some maintained, on the analogy of hydatid cysts, that tumors were caused by spontaneously generated entozoa. Even Dupuytren (1805) and Laënnec (1837) supported the doctrine of parasitism against the sounder views of Fleischmann (1815).

The splendid atlases of the eighteenth and early nineteenth centuries depicted accurately many forms of cancer, and yet in Robert Carswell's "Illustrations of the Elementary Forms of

Disease" (1837) —one of the best—obvious meta-
static nodules in the liver are regarded as transformations of liver substance by cancerous secretion from the blood. Cruveilhier, the leading
pathologist of his time, held the similar view that
the degenerated cancer juice was carried to distant organs by the blood.

The first microscopic illustrations of cancer
are said by Haagensen to be found in Everard
Home's "Short Tract on the Formation of
Tumours," (1830), nine years before the promulgation of the cell theory. In the five microscopic
drawings, however, the cancer cells are labeled
lymph globules, and they are not mentioned
in the text, which expresses the conventional pre-
cellular attitude.

Laënnec, profiting by his compatriot Bichat's
doctrine of the tissues, was able to comprehend
scirrhus, not as a specific kind of tumor, but
merely one in which there was much connective
tissue. He and Bayle were the first to distinguish
cancer of the lung from tuberculosis. Bayle about
this time introduced the word "encephaloid"
for tumors with a brain-like consistency, a term
still used. For both, however, cancer in more
than one organ was merely an evidence of cancerous diathesis.

Although fundamental knowledge of the structure of carcinoma perforce awaited cellular pathology, gross knowledge of special forms could
and did make noteworthy progress. This was
doubtless furthered by the formation of special
societies, such as the Society for Investigating
the Nature and Cure of Cancer, which was
founded in England in 1802 by Baillie, Sims,

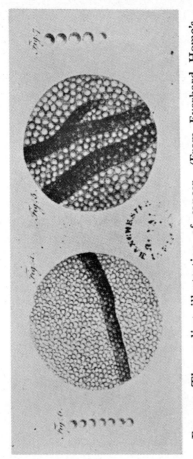

FIG. 17. The earliest illustration of cancer. (From Everhard Home's "Short Tract on the Formation of Tumours.")

Abernethy and others. Various occupational cancers entered the field (chimney sweep's, Pott, 1775; arsenic, John Paris, 1822). The gross pathological knowledge of the great clinicians produced the pictures of cancer of the lung and melanoma (Laënnec, 1815), glioma of the retina (Wardrop, 1809), uterine cancer (von Siebold, 1824), mammary fibroadenoma and chronic cystic mastitis (Astley Cooper, 1829), cancer of the testicle, hydatid, fungoid and scirrhus (Cooper, 1830), malignant disease of the lymphatics (Hodgkin, 1832), the parotid gland (Berard, 1841; McClellan, 1848), the prostate (John Adams, 1851).

The great Rokitansky, with his unfortunate theory of crases, naturally regarded cancer as due to a special crasis, which brought about a local change of the blastema from the blood, the solid blastema producing the fibrous elements, fluid blastema the cellular material. His descriptions of the gross appearance of neoplasms, however, are numerous and accurate.

Thus it becomes obvious that the cell theory was an absolute necessity before the nature of cancer could be comprehended. After its promulgation, histological knowledge of tumors was one of the first lines of advance. But even so, adequate tumor knowledge came slowly. No sooner had Schwann extended Schleiden's cell theory of plants to animal tissue than his master, the great Johannes Müller, applied this knowledge to the study of tumors. In fact, even before Schwann's publication, he had written about the reticular and fasciculate types of carcinoma (1836).

In the same year with Schwann he published "Ueber den feineren Bau und die Formen der krankhaften Geschwulste" (translated in 1840 by Charles West with the title "On the Nature and Structural Characteristics of Cancer," etc.). The plates, many from drawings by Schwann, and statements in the text show that Müller clearly recognized not only cells, their nuclei and nucleoli, but could distinguish various types of tumor histologically and had sound ideas on the nature of neoplasm. "Thus . . . did the examination of morbid structures confirm Schwann's observations . . . of healthy tissues." "The cell is by far the most frequent element of morbid growths." Carcinoma was recognized as not heterologous, arising from the same units of structure as benign tumors, and its microscopic difference from "induration" and ulcer was appreciated. It was regarded as a constitutional disease in the sense that it recurred after removal (i.e., a tendency, not a failure to remove completely), though it was recognized that occasionally true carcinoma was cured by removal. How little of the following sentences needs to be changed today: "The manner in which the carcinomatous dyscarsia becomes developed from a merely local disposition transcends our researches. It can, however, be easily understood that when once cells with a productive tendency have been formed, the reception of the germinal nuclei into the circulation may determine their distribution into some part predisposed to receive them and may thus give rise to the formation of secondary tumors." This is an understanding of tumor metastasis far in advance of any previous doctrine, which had to survive Virchow's erroneous views on the subject before becoming finally established. On the other hand, both Müller and Schwann were infected with the blastema idea of cells within cells as the means of reproduction; they still spoke of "sarcoma" as a benign tumor, and they believed that "microscopic and chemical analysis can never become a means of surgical diagnosis: it were ridiculous to desire it or suppose it practicable" (West's translation).

Noteworthy is *Charles Robin's* (1821-85) "Mémoire sur l'épithélioma du rein" (1855), in which he demonstrated that renal cancer arose from the tubular epithelium, with rupture of the membrana propria by the neoplastic cells to form the solid cancer nodules. Too little known, also, is the work of the Copenhagen pathologist, *Adolph Hannover* (1814-94) who coined the term "epithelioma" (1852), even though he did not recognize the condition's malignant character, and maintained that metastases were produced by cancer cells arriving by way of the blood stream.

While the great Virchow was putting the entire subject of morbid anatomy on a rational basis, his earlier views of malignant disease contained a number of errors. Neoplasms were considered by him to be either homologous (e.g. uterine fibroid, made of tissue belonging to the part) or heterologous (e.g., cancer, where the cells were changed in character). These were terms coined by Lobstein (1829) to indicate tumors that corresponded to or were foreign to the tissue in which they were found. Though

Virchow was the first to solve the great question of thrombosis, secondary cancer nodules were for him not due to emboli, because they often did not occur in the direct line of the circulation, but rather to certain fluids which possess the power of disposing parts to reproduce a mass of the same nature as the original. Again, "an ichorous piece may pass from a cancerous tumor through the lungs without producing any change in them and yet at a more remote point an ichorous collection excites changes of a malignant nature." This is not far distant from such views as Carswell's that have already been referred to. Though Virchow asserted *"omnis cellula e cellula,"* yet he thought a cell might be transformed (cf. metaplasia) and thus that carcinoma started from connective tissue cells.

It remained for his colleague, *Robert Remak* (1815-65), to show that skin cancer arose from skin epithelium and not from connective tissue, a fact proved by the surgeon Thiersch's razor-cut serial sections and extended to epithelial tumors of internal organs by Waldeyer. The nature of metastasis, both by embolism in the lymph and blood channels and by direct extension, was solved by the great anatomist, Waldeyer, not long after. Hansemann's concept (1902) of histological "anaplasia," i.e., that tumor cells become more embryonic in character, was an important addition to the understanding of the nature of cancer.

Knowledge of the causes of cancer, however, progressed but little and of course still awaits a complete answer. The importance of Cohnheim's theory of the activation of dormant embryonic rests (1877) is still to be correctly evaluated; likewise *Hugo Ribbert's* (1855-1920) modification that adult cells might be similarly segregated by the irregular growth of adjacent tissue. Virchow's emphasis on irritation as a cause is warmly upheld today, but is known not to constitute the whole story. External causes of cancer were demonstrated before the end of the nineteenth century among others by: Volkmann (tar and paraffin cancer, 1875); Hürting and Hesse (miner's cancer of the lung, 1879); R. H. Harrison (bilharzia cancer of the bladder, 1889); Rehn (aniline cancer, 1895). Hosts of parasites have been proposed, only to be discredited, but at least it can be said that the problem is being diligently and extensively followed and constantly more facts are being brought to light.

In the present generation the outstanding contributions have been the various studies in experimental cancer: transmissible tumors in animals (Hanau, 1889; Morau, 1894; Leo Loeb, 1901; Jensen, 1903); artificial production of cancer: nematode gastric cancer of rats (Fibiger, 1913), tar cancer of the skin (Yamagiwa and Ichikawa, 1916), cysticercus sarcoma of liver (Bullock and Rohdenburg, 1915), production by cell-free filtrates of viruses (in fowl, Rous; rabbits, Shope; frogs, Lucké); production by chemicals of known composition (Kennaway and others), some of the substances being related to body products such as bile salts and estrogens; hereditary studies by Slye, Little and many others; the effect of roentgen ray and radium on various kinds of neoplastic tissue, manifestations of resistance and adaptation and War-

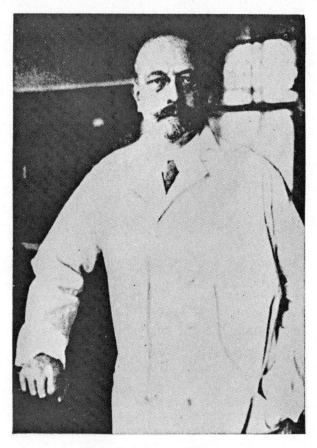

FIG. 18. Johannes Fibiger.
(From an original photograph.)

burg's demonstration of the peculiar fermenta-
tive type of metabolism of the cancer cell. This
condensation into a single sentence of the
contributions of the present century, fitting perhaps in a historical presentation, should not
obscure the truly remarkable progress that they
represent. As in other fields of medicine, the past
100 years have added more to our knowledge of
cancer than have all the preceding centuries, and
the accumulation of cancer facts is progressing
more rapidly today than in any previous generation. While the cause of cancer, in the sense
of the precise mechanism that makes the normal
cell become cancerous, still remains unknown,
each decade now sees a noteworthy increase in
the formidable array of evidence as to the nature
of the condition. It is not presumptuous, then,
to hope that adequate knowledge as to its essential cause, and therefore probably as to its control, will not be long in forthcoming.

EPILOGUE

THOUGH the mind still experiences difficulty, and probably always will to a greater or less degree, in functioning without dogmatism, nevertheless it can be fairly said that the day of philosophic systems of disease largely unsupported by evidence is definitely past. For most of the past century, pathology has been modestly content to observe and experiment, base conclusions and theories as far as possible on facts, and wait when the facts are insufficient. Wrong observations and mistaken deductions continue—some are quickly corrected, others doubtless await correction by our successors; but the proper scientific method of progress, let us hope, has been established for good and all. A system of medicine not based on pathology is indeed difficult to contemplate.

And what of the future? Is Pathology, which on the anatomical side at least entered into its heyday in the middle of the last century, to be regarded as having made its major contribution and to be put aside for disciplines more effective toward the conquest of disease? The answer probably depends largely on the point of view and kind of activity indulged in by its followers. Interpreted as a synonym for pathological anatomy, pathology would indeed seem to have yielded its most important secrets, in the same sense that normal anatomy had accomplished its main task over a century ago. Even from this restricted standpoint, however, not only is there still much to be learned in the absolute sense, but also with each new development of other contributory sciences, the well-tilled field of morbid anatomy must be gone over again, often with surprising discoveries. The myocardium, for instance, is still awaiting such treatment when electrocardiography has been sufficiently developed.

According to the wider definition of pathology (the study of the nature of disease in its functional as well as structural changes) that has been used in this booklet, the future of pathology is only limited by the ability of its devotees to adapt themselves to changing points of view, methods of attack and accumulations of new knowledge. The task is no easy one and each decade brings a more complex field to be mastered. But a similar problem faces the scientific clinician, whose field logically overlaps or is often almost identical with that of the pathologist. Essential differences of training and emphasis will and should always remain (see A. E. Cohn's thoughtful essays on "Medicine, Science and Art," 1931) ; but it is becoming increasingly clear that the serious student of disease, whether working primarily in the pathological laboratory or in the clinic, must be equipped to study or direct the study of his problem by physical, chemical, mathematical and experimental methods, as well as by the older methods of anatomy or bedside study, as the case may be. This should not be regarded as encroaching on the fields of the biophysicist or biochemist any more than is their activity an encroachment when they study pathological as well as normal conditions. Helpful partnerships should often be resorted to; but even without them the field is large enough for both.

Here as elsewhere history often repeats itself for those who can adapt the story to new, changed conditions, so that even this short sketch may perhaps aid some in forecasting the future. At least it should afford some information for those who wish to have a proper background for their life's work, as well as attempting to tell an interesting story to those concerned with man's struggle with disease.

THE WORD "PATHOLOGY"

AS EVERY medical student early learns, or should learn, the word "Pathology" is derived from πάθος, suffering or disease, and λόγος, a discourse or study. It therefore might be thought a more suitable name for our profession than "medicine," which presumably conquered through its euphemistic emphasis on the idea of healing contained in its derivation. Pathology, however, becoming more restricted in its definition has come to indicate the study of the nature of disease, or of the structural and functional changes produced by disease. Some English-speaking countries have even confused Pathology with one of its branches, pathological anatomy, though in France and Germany the word used with various adjectives, such as "internale," "externale," "spezielle," becomes synonymous with medicine and surgery.

The word can be traced as far back as Galen, who, for instance, says (according to a translation kindly made by Dr. W. B. McDaniel, 2nd, from "Opera Omnia," Kühn's edition, volume 19, p. 458): "In the pathological department of medicine is included both general and localized disease, also its causes, signs and differences," and again (Vol. 14, p. 689) "parts of medicine . . . are aetiology and pathology."

I have not been able to find the word used in the Hippocratic Corpus or in other pre-Galenic authors. Mr. A. K. Borman, Research Librarian at the University of Pennsylvania, has found for me a fifth century use of the word in J. Stobaeus', "Eclogorum physicarum et ethicarum libri duo" (Ed. T. Gaisford, Oxon., 1850) ; also in an eleventh century manuscript in the Bibliothèque Nationale (Quicherat, Addenda Lexicis Latinis, Paris, 1862). Here it is defined as *ratio passionis,* or the nature of disease. Hippocrates, to be sure, stressed what might be called the general pathology or picture of disease, above diagnosis, for example, but this concept was included in his term "Prognostic." The nearest to "pathology" that I can find in the Hippocratic Corpus is $\pi\alpha\theta\acute{\eta}\mu\alpha$ (symptom), as in line 10 of "Prognostic."

From the sixteenth century on, the word was in frequent use, and in much the same sense as we use it today. We have seen Fernel's use of it as a subdivision of his "Universa Medicina," while Jacques Guillemeau (English translation, 1597) states "Pathologia treatethe of the cause and occasione of the sicknesses."

EARLY CHAIRS OF PATHOLOGY AND PATHOLOGIC ANATOMY

THE earliest independent chair of pathologic anatomy is usually said to be that founded at Strasbourg for J. F. D. Lobstein in 1819. Even this, however, was temporarily combined in 1821 with the chair of Internal Medicine. Chairs of pathology had of course existed for a much longer time; but, as we have just seen, this meant something very different from what is meant by Pathology today, and they were usually combined with chairs of other subjects. Lobstein himself had been Professor of Pathology at Strasbourg in 1783, where from 1674-1701 Marcus Mappas had been Professor of Botany and Pathology. F. Wieger's "Geschichte der Medicin . . . in Strassburg" (Strassburg, 1885), gives a long list of such professorships in various combinations.

Similarly, von Bergen was Professor of Pathology and Therapy at Frankfurt in 1744; and the well-known Christian Gottlieb Ludwig, after being made Professor of Medicine, Anatomy and Surgery, became Professor of Pathology at Leipsic in 1755. His son, Christian Friedrich, held the same chair there in 1796. Other eighteenth century professors of pathology (not necessarily the first in their universities) were: 1767, Tübingen, C. F. Jaeger (combined with clinical medicine); 1794, Altdorf, J. C. G. Ackermann (combined with therapy); 1794, Parma, G. A. D.

Tommasini (combined with physiology) ; 1798, Paris, Ph. Pinel (internal pathology or medicine) ; 1798, Würzburg, A. Roeschlaub (combined with medical clinic).

In the early nineteenth century we find: 1803, Montpellier, J. B. T. Baumes (in 1824 this was restricted to Pathologie Médicale) ; 1804, Wilna. J. F. Frank, 1806; Josephs Akademie, Vienna, Joseph Ritter von Scherer (pathologic anatomy and physiology; this is the earliest chair of pathologic anatomy that I have found) ; 1810, Vienna, P. K. Hartmann (General Pathology, and Materia Medics) ; 1815, Marburg, S. C. Lucae (Pathology and Therapy) ; 1815, Leipsic, F. A. B. Puchelt (Pathology and Therapy).

The increasing emphasis on the new and exact study of pathologic anatomy seems to have been responsibile for the many full-time chairs that were created shortly after Lobstein's appointment. The influence of this trend is still to be seen in the persistence of professorships of "pathologic anatomy" alone or in combination with other titles such as "general pathology" or "functional pathology," especially in Germany and the Latin countries. It is only in the English-speaking countries that most schools use the broader and more correct term "pathology" to designate this chair.

The University College, London, appointed J. F. Meckel Professor of Morbid and Comparative Anatomy in 1827 but he never took up his duties. The next year Sir Robert Carswell was nominated, but he did not assume the position till 1831, as he was in Paris working on material for his Atlas. The chair of Morbid Anatomy was held by G. S. Pattison from 1828 to 1831. In

1832, Vienna appointed John Wagner (who had been prosecutor since 1830) *ausserordentlicher* Professor of pathologic anatomy. He was succeeded on his death the next year by the celebrated Rokitansky. Another important chair was that of the University of Paris (1836) founded by Dupytren for his pupil, Cruveilhier. In Berlin, the chair of pathologic anatomy was not established until 1856 when the already great Virchow was brought from Würzburg.

In the United States the first chair was created at Harvard, when in 1847 J. B. S. Jackson was appointed Professor of Pathological Anatomy, a position that he held until 1879, his successors being R. H. Fitz and, in 1892, W. T. Councilman. At the University of Pennsylvania, James Tyson was made Professor of Pathologic Anatomy in 1867, and at the College of Physicians and Surgeons in New York Francis Delafield, who had been Adjunct Professor since 1875, was made full professor in 1882. The change to "Professor of Pathology" at Pennsylvania was made with Simon Flexner's appointment in 1899, presumably in recognition of the broader significance of the shorter title; at Harvard, the older form persists, but it is rarely found today in American medical schools. Well before the close of the nineteenth century, every self-respecting medical school had an independent chair for this important subject.

CHRONOLOGICAL LIST OF PATHOLOGIC MILESTONES

As it has been impossible to include mention of many pathological conditions, even of major importance, in the text of this small book, the following list has been compiled to indicate important events in the history of the causes of, nature of, and changes produced by disease. It obviously makes no pretense at completeness or complete accuracy. In many cases the authority does not need to be given, in some it cannot be traced. Where the honor of a first description has been shared by more than one author, the others have been included in brackets with their significant dates.

Ca. 2160-1788 B.C.   Papyrus fragments dealing with diseases of women and cattle.

Ca. 1600 B.C.   Edwin Smith Papyrus noted fractures, dislocations, wounds and their results (e.g., paralysis from brain injury; infection of wound of breast), diseases of the eye, tumors, etc.

Ca. 1550 B.C.   Ebers Papyrus: coryza, dysentery, mastoiditis, diseases of bones and joints, tumors, cysts, parasitic diseases, abscess, many diseases of the eye, gastrointestinal tract and female genitalia.

Ca. 1000 B.C.   Bubonic plague (?) (emerods and mice) (I Samuel 6: 4, 5). Also "the itch" (Deut. 28: 27).

Ca. 650 B.C.   *Archilochus* mentioned phymata (probably abscesses, tubercles, as well as true tumors). (See Gurlt.)

Ca. 650 B.C.   Library of Assurbanipal contained reference to monsters, epilepsy (*Hammurabi,* 2080 B.C.), paralytic stroke, falling sickness, leprosy, gonorrhea, rheumatism, heart disease, scabies, pediculosis, etc.

Ca. 600 B.C.   Lex regia (postmortem cesarean section).

***Ca.* 500 b.c.** *Susruta's* "Samhita": disease of rats connected with contagion (bubonic plague?) (Bhagavata Purana) ; urinary calculi, cholera, association of mosquitoes (*masakas*) with malaria (?) (*Vishama-jwara*), diabetes (?) (*Madhumeha*) ; etc.

***Ca.* 425 b.c.** *Thucydides'* account of the plague of Athens (bubonic?).

***Ca.* 400 b.c.** *Hippocrates:* disease due to dyscrasia of the humors. Good pictures of phthisis, pleurisy, pneumonia, cirrhosis, tetanus, sore-throat (quinsy? diphtheria?), cancer, mumps, erysipelas, and many other diseases.

***Ca.* 250 b.c.** *Erasistratus* attributed disease of a part to plethora; connected ascites with hardness of liver. Probably first to do necropsies to determine cause of death.

***Ca.* 56 b.c.** *Lucretius'* "De natura rerum": descriptions of epilepsy (Bk. iii), the Plague of Athens (Bk. vi) ; Evolution of Man (Bk. v).

***Ca.* 25 a.d.** *Celsus'* "De re medicina": nasal polyps, caries, enlarged tonsils, pneumonia, cancer of the mouth, inguinal hernia, appendicitis, splenomegaly, skin diseases (chancre and chancroid). Gives four classical signs of inflammation (Bk. iii).

***Ca.* 100** *Rufus of Ephesus* (Paul of Aegina's translation) gave clear description of pneumonic plague and is said by Littré to mention buboes.

Archigenes recognized cancer of the breast in men and women.

Metrodora described diseases of the womb (earliest medical treatise by a woman?)

Soranos: metritis, uterine scleromata, leucorrhea, metrorrhagia, apoplexy (due to mucus in cerebral ventricles).

***Ca.* 150** *Aretaeus:* leprosy, diabetes, tetanus, diphtheria (ulcera syriaca), dysenteric ulcers, relation of anasarca to heart disease, asthma, cerebral and spinal paralysis.

Ca. 170   *Galen* added fifth cardinal sign of inflammation; classified tumors and fevers. Developed experimental pathology.

302   *Bishop Eusebius* described a Syrian epidemic of smallpox.

580   Quinsy *(esquinancie)* mentioned in St. Denis chronicle.

590   Epidemic of ergotism in France.

Ca. 643   *Paul of Aegina* described carbuncle (anthrax).

Ca. 900.   *Rhazes:* First clear description of smallpox and measles. Observed spina ventosa, and the parasitic nature of guinea worm (Avicenna, Canon III, 2, Ch. 21).

Ca. 1000   *Avicenna's* "Canon" became the universal medical textbook. Invisible animals (waterborne) as cause of disease; differentiation of hemolytic from obstructive jaundice. Arabic doctrine of laudable pus.

1004   *Baronius* described epidemic of suffocative angina (laryngeal diphtheria?) in Rome.

1087   *Anglo-Saxon Chronicle* mentioned typhus fever (?).

Ca. 1100   *Avenzoar* described cancer of the esophagus and stomach, serous pericarditis. Was the first to describe the itch mite. (Aristotle; Bonomo, 1687; Wichmann, 1786; Renucci, 1834).

13th cent.   Spread of leprosy through Europe reached its height.

1200   *Ruggiero Frugardi* of Palermo and Salerno in "Practica chirurgiae" recognized a relationship between sponges and seaweed (iodine) and goiter. Also observed cancer and (possibly) syphilis.

1231 *Frederick* ii's edict favoring human dissection.

1240 *Gilbertus Anglicus* recognized contagiosity of smallpox ("Compendium medicinae").

1250 *Joinville* described scurvy ("mal d'ost") in Louis ix's troops at Cairo.

1252 *Bruno* avoided pus in healing of wounds (also Hugh of Lucca, Theodoric and Henri de Mondeville).

1275 *Guglielmo da Saliceto* mentioned "durities in renibus" and renal dropsy. Performed autopsies. ("Summa conservationis.")

1286 *Salimbene of Parma's* "Chronicon" reported autopsy on case of plague at Cremona.

1296 *Lanfranchi* differentiated cancer of the breast from hypertrophy, and arterial from venous hemorrhage.

1302 First medico-legal autopsy by *Bartolomeo da Varignana.*

1319 First criminal prosecution for body snatching.

1341 *Gentile da Foligno* performed public dissection in Padua. Described gallstones. (*Marcello Donato*, 1586.)

1348-50 The Black Death (Boccaccio, 1353; Guy de Chauliac, 1363).

1363 *Guy de Chauliac* classified abscesses; good description of leprosy.

1374-75 Dancing mania (chorea) in Germany and France.

Ca. 1376 *John of Arderne* described "passio iliaca" (appendicitis ?).

1404 First public dissection in Vienna.

1410 Autopsy on Pope Alexander v by *Pietro d'Argelata.*

1414 Coqueluche epidemic (influenza ?) in France.

Ca. 1460 *Savonarola* noted results of contracted pelvis in labor.

Ca. 1470 *Bartolommeo Montagnana* known to have dissected at least fourteen bodies.

1485   Sweating sickness (influenza?) (miliary fever?) appeared in England. (See Caius' "Boke," 1552.)

1492   *Schedel:* diphtheria epidemic in Nuremberg.

1495-1500 Syphilis overran Europe (Kaiser Maximilian's edict against blasphemers includes first printed mention of "pösen plattern," Aug. 7, 1495).

1497   *Alessandro Benedetti* described gallstones and malposition of the heart. Upheld need for autopsies.

1501   Morbus Hungaricus (camp fever, typhus ?) overran camps in Europe.

1506   *Benivieni's* posthumous "De abditis causis morborum," is first collection of autopsy reports.

1510   Influenza pandemic in Europe (recurred four times in each succeeding century and in 1917).

1521   *Berengario da Carpi's* "Commentaria" cited his performance of many autopsies.

1530   *Fracastoro's* poem, "Syphilis."

1532   *Niccolò Massa:* visceral gummata (*"materiae albae viscosae"*); syphilis as cause of mental disease.

1533   Autopsy of double human monster (San Domingo).

1535-36 *Jacques Cartier* observed epidemic of scurvy in his fleet.

1536   *Cardano* gave early account of typhus (*morbus pulicaris*) in "De malo recent. med. usu."

1546   *Fracastoro's* treatise "De morbis contagiosis."

Ca. 1550 Epidemics of leprosy and chorea largely disappeared from Europe.

1552   *Matthaeus Friedrich* said to have written the first treatise on alcoholism.

1553   *Ingrassia* described chickenpox (named and elaborated by Heberden, 1767).

1554   *Fernel's* "Universa medicina," included a treatise on .pathology. Described appendicitis ("iliac passion") in Bk. VI.

Johannes Lange: First published description of chlorosis (*morbus virgineus*) ("Epist. med.").

1559 *Colombo's* "De re anatomica" (Bk. XV) (calculi in kidneys, ureter, bladder, lungs, liver, portal vein, gall bladder, colon, hemorrhoidal veins; abscesses of vagina, heart; tumors of mediastinum).

1567 Posthumous publication of *Paracelsus'* account of miner's phthisis ("Von der Bergsucht").

1573 *Volcher Coiter* described cerebrospinal meningitis (Vieusseux, Danielson and Mann, 1805).

1575 *Paré* said to have described carbon-monoxide poisoning (?).

Baillou described laryngeal croup (?) (*morbus incognitus*). ("Consiliorum," Bk. III, Obs. 89).

1578 *Baillou* described whooping cough under general term "quinta." (Epid. et Ephemer., Bk. II) (Alberti, 1728).

Garnerus observed huge spleen and liver at autopsy (splenomyelogenous leucemia?).

1580 Scurvy in Drake's sailors on his voyage around the world.

1584 *Scribonius* described alcaptonuria (*Garrod*).

1591 *d'Acosta* described mountain sickness ("Hist. nat. y moral de las Indias").

1598 *Fedeli* established need for autopsies in poisoning cases.

1602 *F. Plater* described cretinism ("Praxeos"). (See also Paracelsus' "Posthumus Opera," 1603; Heufer, 1657; Curling, 1850, absent thyroid.)

1605 Autopsies of scurvy cases at Ste. Croix (Champlain's voyages).

1606 *Cober's* "Observationes castrenses" noted relation between lice and morbus Hungaricus.

1607 *Fabricius Hildanus* established three degrees of burns ("De combustionibus").

1614 *Felix Plater* described first case of thymic death in infancy (in *Bonet's* "Sepulchretum"). Observed sublingual calculus, gigantism, brain tumor, cystic liver and kidneys.

1619 *Fabricius Hildanus* connected psychoses with head injuries.

1623-25 Purpuric fever in Britain.

1624 *Antoine Saporta's* posthumous "De tumoribus" cited case of aortic aneurysm diagnosed in 1554.

1625 *Michael Doering* described scarlet fever. (*Sennert*, 1619, probably confused scarlet fever and measles.)

1628 *Harvey* "De motu cordis" first permitted adequate views of pathologic anatomy and physiology.

1629 London bills of mortality begin to specify causes of death (*John Graunt*) (first published, 1592).

1630 *Thuillier* related ergotism to poisoning by corn smut.

1632 *Severino's* "De recondita abscessuum natura" first treatise on surgical pathology, and among the first illustrated medical books.

1640 Coup de barre (yellow fever ?) at *Guadeloupe* (Dutertre, 1647-48).

1641 *Tulp's* "Observationum medicarum" has good description of cancer of the bladder, spina bifida, etc. (Bk. III). Bronchial cast described as a vein (Bk. II).
Bontius' posthumously published description of beri-beri ("De med. indorum"). (Also *Tulp*, 1652; *Malcolmson*, 1835.)

1642 Baillou's posthumous "Liber de rheumatismo," first use of word.

1647 *William Harvey* first to describe heart rupture.

1650 *Glisson* described rickets ("Tract. de rachitide") . (*Daniel Whistler*, 1645.)
Franciscus Sylvius related tubercles to phthisis
and recognized tuberculosis of lymph nodes.

1656 *Pierre Borel* "Historiarum . . . Cent. iv," first
work applying microscopy to. medicine
(erythrocytes, acarus scabiei, gastric fistula).

1658 *Wepfer* demonstrated relation of cerebral
hemorrhage to apoplexy.
Kircher attributed plague to a contagium
animatum ("Scrutinium pestis") . Early use
of microscopy in "Ars lucis et umbrae"
(1646) .

1659 *Willis* described the military epidemic of
typhoid of 1643. Also described and named
puerperal fever.

1665 The Great Plague of London (*Defoe*, 1722) .

1666 *Malpighi* described enlarged lymph nodes and
spleen (Hodgkin's disease ?), in "De vis-
cerum structura"; also aortic sclerosis and
osteomyelitis.

1667 *Willis* described the general paralysis of the
insane.
Swammerdam observed that fetal lungs float
only after respiration has been established
("Tract. de resp.," Ch. 3) .

1667-69 *Giovanni Riva* started a society for pathological discussion, also a pathological museum.

1668-72 Epidemic of dysentery in England described
by *Sydenham* and *Morton*.

1668 *Redi's* experiments disproved doctrine of
spontaneous generation.

1669 *Lower* produced edema by ligating veins
("Tract. de corde") .
Vincent Ketelaer described sprue ("De aphthis
nostratibus") . (Also *Hillary*, 1759.)

1670 *Theodore Kerckring's* "Spicilegium ana-

tomicum"   (i.a., described the valvulae con-
niventes).

1673 *Willis* described sweet urine of diabetes mellitus ("De medic. operat.").
Dekkers described albuminuria in his "Exercit.
pract." (Ch. VIII).

1676 *Sydenham* identified and named scarlet fever,
and differentiated it from measles.
Wiseman first to describe joint tuberculosis
(*Tumor albus*).

1677 Publication of *Glisson's* doctrine of irritability
of the tissues.

1679 *Bonet's* "Sepulchretum anatomicum" (contains
first observations of many pathological conditions, including pituitary cyst).

1680 *Zambeccari* studied effect of excision of viscera
in animals ("Experimente intorno," etc.,
quoted by Morgagni, Animad. Anat., II,
Obs. 24).

1683 *Leeuwenhoek* described and depicted bacteria.
Tyson dissected intestinal parasites of man.
Sydenham described acute gout ("Tract. de
podagra").

1685 *Willis* described condition now known as
myasthenia gravis (*Erb*, 1878).
John Brown of Southwark described and depicted cirrhosis of liver ("glandulous")
(*Phil. Tr. Roy. Soc. Abr.*, 3: 248).

1686 *Sydenham* described chorea minor ("Schedula
monitoria").

1688 *Stephen Blankaart's* "Anatomia practica," an
important pathological collection (first to
recognize cardiac polyp as a postmortem
change).

1689 *Richard Morton's* "Phthisiologia" (crude tubercles and aposthemes or cavities, tracheo-
bronchial node involvement).

1691   *Peter Middleton's* autopsy on Governor Slaughter of New York.

1693   *Baglivi* described heat stroke in Rome, also intestinal and lymph changes of typhoid fever (*febris mesenterica*) (1696).

1698   *Stahl's* treatise, "De venae portae" emphasized plethora as a cause of disease.
       Mangetus described disseminated miliary tuberculosis.

1700   *Ramazzini's* "De morbis artificium" the first book on occupational diseases.

1701-16 *Frederick Ruysch's* "Thesauri anatomici" signalized permanent collections of pathologic specimens.

1702   *Stahl* described lachrymal fistula.

1705   *Brisseau* established before French Academy of Sciences that clouding of the lens was the cause of cataract (*Rolfink*, 1656).
       Vieussens' treatise elucidated cardiac pathology (mitral stenosis, aortic insufficiency, secondary passive congestion, bounding pulse).

1709   *Boerhaave* described heat-stroke as "insolation."

1711   *Heister* performed autopsy on case of appendicitis.

1713   Botulism said to have been described as sausage poisoning by *Onoldini*.
       Berlin Theatrum Anatomicum founded.

1715   *Vieussens* described and depicted mitral stenosis.

1718   *Pierre Dionis* described tubal pregnancy.
       Friedrich Hoffmann's "Medicina rationalis systematica" included many first or early descriptions.

1719   *Morgagni* described visceral syphilis.

1724   *Boerhaave* described rupture of the esophagus in Baron de Wassenaer, and fatal mediastinal tumor (1728).

1728 *Lancisi's* posthumous "De motu cordis et aneurysmatibus": vegetative endocarditis, luetic nature of aortic aneurysm, first description of cardiac syphilis (*aneurysma gallicum*).

1733 *Stephen Hales* produced edema experimentally by injecting water into veins.

1734 *Werlhof:* the hemorrhagic disease now known as purpura hemorrhagica.
John Atkins: sleeping sickness in Guinea.

1735 *Gaspar Casál's* description of pellagra (*mal de la rosa*), published 1762. (*Thiéry,* J. de Med., 1755; named by *Frapolli,* 1771.)

1736 *William Douglas:* first appearance of scarlet fever in New England, and first unmistakable description.
John Freke: myositis ossificans.

1737 *Huxham* differentiated ship fever (malignant typhus) clinically from "slow nervous fever" (typhoid).

1740 *Friedrich Hoffmann* described rubella.
Astruc's "Diseases Incident to Women" portrayed scirrhus as a lymphatic change and cancer as a development of scirrhus. Also wrote "Tractatus pathologicus" (1743).

1741 *John Mitchell* wrote on yellow fever in America. (Colden, 1743; *Lining,* 1753; *Currie,* 1792; *Carey,* 1793; named by *Griffith Hughes,* 1750.)

1743 *J. Z. Platner* affirmed tuberculous nature of humpback (*Hippocrates, Galen, Delpech* [1816]).

1745 *Thomas Cadwalader* in "An Essay on the West India Dry Gripes" described lead poisoning (*Huxham,* 1739; *Nikander,* 2nd cent. A.D.). Also described a case of osteomalacia.

1746 *Fauchard's* description of pyorrhea alveolaris in second edition of "Le chirurgien dentiste" (*Riggs,* 1876).

1748 *Fothergill* gave first authoritative description of diphtheria.

La Fosse studied the pathology of glanders.

1749 *Sénac's* "Traité de la structure du coeur."

1753 *Lind's* "Treatise of the Scurvy" established its control by lemon juice.

1755 *Haller's* "Opuscula pathologica" included a case of "stone heart."

1757 *William Hunter* described arteriovenous aneurysm. Wrote on emphysema.

1758 *de Haen* first to perform autopsies routinely before students (Vienna).

1760 *Patrick Russell:* Aleppo button (endemic ulcer).

1761 *Morgagni's* "De sedibus et causis morborum" inaugurated modern gross pathology and described many *nova.*

Auenbrugger's "Inventum novum" announced percussion and correlated clinical, experimental and postmortem findings.

Hamilton observed orchitis in mumps.

1763 *R. A. Vogel* described paranoia.

1765 *Francis Home:* the false membrane of diphtheritic croup.

Sagar related hoof and mouth disease of cattle to aphthous fever in man.

1767 *Heberden* distinguished chickenpox from smallpox. Also observed nyctalopia (*Nettleship,* 1909).

George Baker connected Devonshire colic and colica pictonum with lead poisoning.

George Armstrong: congenital pyloric stenosis.

1768 *Heberden's* classic description of angina pectoris. (See death of Earl of Clarendon, 1674.)

Whytt described tuberculous meningitis (*Papavoine,* 1830; *Lediberder,* 1837).

1769 *Cullen's* "Synopsis nosologiae methodicac" guided medical thought for a half century.

1770   *John Rutty* described relapsing fever ("A Chronological History, etc.").
        William Hunter described retroverted uterus.
        Cotugno described sciatica; related albuminuria to dropsy.

1771   *John Hunter's* "Natural History of the Human Teeth."

1773   *Charles White's* "Phlegmasia alba Dolens."
        Fothergill described facial neuralgia.

1775   *Pott's* discovery of chimney sweep's (scrotal) cancer—the first to demonstrate an external cause for cancer.

1776   *Plenck's* "Doctrina" classified skin diseases.
        Dobson first to note sugar in diabetic urine.

1777-79 *Eduard Sandifort's* "Observationes anatomico-pathologicae."

1779   *Bylon of Java* described dengue (*Benjamin Rush,* 1780).
        Pott related spinal caries to paralyses.

1785   *John Hunter* elucidated the collateral circulation of aneurysm by experiments on stags' antlers.

1786   *John Hunter's* "Treatise on Venereal Disease."
        Parry first described exophthalmic goiter (*Flajani,* 1800; *Graves,* 1835; *Basedow,* 1840).
        Fourcroy and *Thourlt* discovered adipocere in human remains.

1788   *Pitcairn* lectured on the relation of rheumatism to heart disease.

1789   *John Hunter* described intussusception.
        Matthew Baillie observed ovarian dermoid cysts.

1791   *Soemmerring* described achondroplasia.

1793   Yellow fever epidemic in Philadelphia; *Rush* noted prevalence of mosquitoes.
        Benjamin Bell differentiated between gonorrhea and syphilis.

Baillie's "Morbid Anatomy," first systematic modern treatise on pathology.

1794 *John Hunter's* "Treatise on the Blood, Inflammation and Gunshot Wounds."

Dalton described color blindness (*Mem. Lit. & Phil. Soc.*, 1798) .

Johann Peter Frank defined diabetes insipidus.

1795 *Baillie* described endocarditis.

1797 *Wollaston* isolated uric acid from gouty joints.

1798 *John Haslam* described general paralysis of the insane (*Willis*, 1667) .

1799-1800 *Bichat's* "Traité des membranes" established tissue pathology, paving way from organic to cellular pathology.

1801 *Rush* relation between diseased teeth and distant disease (theory of focal infection) .

Young described astigmatism.

1802 *Laënnec* described peritonitis.

1803 *Alois Vetter's* "Aphorismen aus der pathologischen Anatomie," based on several thousand autopsies.

J. C. Otto established hemophilia as an inherited clinical entity.

Thomas Winterbottom gave earliest account of African sleeping sickness (Kondee) .

1804 *Scarpa* described arteriosclerosis.

1806 *Laënnec* described melanoma and differentiated cancer of the lung from tuberculosis.

Corvisart's "Essai sur les maladies . . . du coeur . . ." (cardiac hypertrophy, dilatation and fibrosis) .

1808 *Cayol* observed bronchiectasis.

1810 *Bayle* emphasized relation of tubercle to phthisis ("Recherches sur la phthisie pulmonaire") . (*Stark*, 1788.)

1812 *Wells* described cardiac changes of rheumatic fever (*Tr. Soc. Impr. M. & Chir. Knowl.*) .

Wood described neuroma (*Edin. M. & S. J.*) .

1815 *Hodgson's* description of aortic aneurysm ("Engravings intended," etc.).

1817 *Parkinson's* "Essay on the Shaking Palsy."
Romberg's thesis on achondroplasia, "De Rachitide Congenita."

1817-26 *Meckel* systematized human anomalies.

1818 *De Riemer* introduced frozen section technique.
Rayer's thesis on History of Pathology, first on this subject.

1819 *Lobstein* first professor of pathologic anatomy, as an independent chair (Strasbourg).
Laënnec's "Auscultation médiate," clarified tuberculosis, pneumothorax, cirrhosis, and diseases of the chest, endocarditis, aneurysms.
Bostock described hay fever (*Botallus*, 1565; *Binninger*, 1673).

1822 *Etienne Geoffroy St. Hilaire's* "Monstruosités humaines."
John Paris discovered arsenic cancer in man and animals ("Pharmacologia").
James Jackson described alcoholic neuritis (*New Eng. M. & S. J.*).

1824 *Bertin* differentiated concentric and eccentric cardiac hypertrophy ("Traité des mal. du coeur").
Selligue's invention of achromatic microscope paved way for cellular pathology (*Chevalier*, 1830).

1825 *Bouillaud* described and localized lesion of aphasia. (*Arch. gén. de méd.*).
Andral and *Louis* described tuberculous peritonitis ("Rech. sur la phthisie").

1826-27 *Rayer's* classification of skin diseases based largely on pathology (*Hebra*, 1845).

1827 *Bright* associated chronic renal disease with dropsy and albuminuria with apoplectiform seizures ("Reports of Medical Cases").

Adams described heart block (*Dublin Hosp. Rep.*). (*Gerbezius*, 1719; *Morgagni*, 1761; *Spens*, 1793; *Stokes*, 1846.)

Hutin described spinal cord changes in locomotor ataxia (*Charcot*).

1829　*Horner's* "Treatise on Pathologic Anatomy," the first published in America on this subject.

Louis' "Recherches . . . sur la gastro-entérite" portrayed intestinal, lymphatic and splenic lesions in typhoid fever.

Recamier described invasion of veins and used term "metastasis" (cerebral) in breast cancer ("Recherches sur le traitement du cancer").

1829-42　*Cruveilhier's* "Anatomie pathologique du corps humain," the peak of pathologic illustration (gastric ulcer, etc.).

1830　*Everard Home's* "Short Tract" gave first microscopic illustrations of cancer.

Steinheim described tetany (*Litt. Ann. d. Ges. Heilk.*).

1832　*Hodgkin's* "Morbid Appearances of the Absorbent Glands and the Spleen" established the condition now known as Hodgkin's disease.

Corrigan described aortic regurgitation (*Edinb. M. & S. J.*). (*Vieussens*, 1686; *Cowper*, 1705; *Hodgkin*, 1827).

1833　*Lobstein:* osteopsathyrosis and arteriosclerosis ("Traité de pathologie").

1834　*Horner* demonstrated nature of rice water stools in cholera.

1835　*Cruveilhier:* multiple sclerosis ("Anat. Path.," livraison 38, pl. 5).

1835-36　*Owen* discovered trichina spiralis (*London Med. Gaz.*).

1836　*Charles Bell* described facial palsy (*Tr. Roy. Soc. Edin.*).

Bright: acute yellow atrophy of liver (*Guy's Hosp. Rep.*). (*Morgagni,* 1762; named by Rokitansky, 1843.)

Cruveilhier, holder of first chair of pathology in Paris, demonstrated blood changes in pyemia.

1836-40 *Hodgkin's* "Morbid Anatomy of the Serous and Mucous Membranes."

1836 *Bouillaud* connected acute articular rheumatism with inflammation of the pericardium, endocardium, and "internal membrane of blood vessels" (*"Nouvelles recherches"*).

Gerhard differentiated typhoid from typhus fever (*Am. J. M. Sc.*).

1837 *Rayer* established contagiousness of glanders.

Schönlein described peliosis rheumatica (*Allg. u. sp. Path. u. Therap.*).

1838 *Johannes Müller's* "Ueber den feineren Bau und die Formen der krankhaften Geschwülsten" first established histologic differences of tumors.

Carswell's "Atlas of Pathologic Anatomy."

Ricord established the independence of lues and gonorrhea and outlined three stages of lues ("Traité pratique").

George Rees observed hyperglycemia in diabetes mellitus (*Guy's Hosp. Rep.*). (*F. Ambrosioni,* 1835.)

1839 *Schwann's* cell theory of animal structure ("Mikroskopische Untersuchungen").

Magendie demonstrated fatal anaphylaxis in rabbits. (Observed by Jenner, 1798.)

S. D. Gross' "Elements of Pathologic Anatomy" covering first regular course given in the United States.

Schönlein discovered the fungus of favus (*Müller's Arch.*).

1840 *Heine* described infantile paralysis ("Beobachtungen").

Henle's essay on Miasms and Contagia promulgated germ theory of disease (in "Path. Untersuchungen").

1842-43 *O. W. Holmes:* contagiousness of puerperal fever. (*Malouin,* 1746; *Semmelweiss,* 1847.)

1842-46 *Rokitansky's* "Lehrbuch der pathologischen Anatomie" (cardiac anomalies).

1843 *Andral's* "Essai d'hématologie pathologique" depicts the blood in disease (spontaneous and secondary anemia).
Julius Vogel's atlas, "Icones Histologiae Pathologicae."
Henderson distinguished relapsing from typhus fever (*Obermaier,* 1873).

1844 New York Pathological Society founded, oldest existing independent society of its kind.

1845 *Virchow* described leucemia (*Neue Notizen*). (*J. Hughes Bennett,* 1845 and 1851.)
Lebert's atlas, "Physiologie pathologique."

1846 *Virchow* elucidated mechanism of thrombosis and embolism (new terms).
London Pathological Society founded.

1846-53 *Henle's* "Handbuch der rationellen Pathologie."

1847 *Virchow* founded *Arch. f. path. Anat. u. Physiol. u. f. klin. Medizin.*

1848 Actinomycosis discovered in man by *B. von Langenbeck* (quoted by J. Israel, *Virch. Arch.,* 74: 15, 1878).

1849 *Thomas Addison* described pernicious (idiopathic) anemia (*Combe,* 1822). Also "Addison's disease" of the adrenals (Monograph, 1855), beginning study of endocrinology.
Claude Bernard produced experimental glycosuria by puncture of the fourth ventricle. (*Compt. rend. Soc. de biol.*)

1850 *E. Dittrich* made first real study of sclerosis of the pulmonary artery. (Said to have been described by *Andral,* 1829; J. Hope, 1833.)

Bacteriology in relation to disease, inaugurated by *Davaine's* discovery of anthrax bacillus ("Traité des entozaires").

Chatin demonstrated the relation between insufficient iodine intake and simple goitre.

Curling connected absent thyroid with myxedematous state (*Med. Chir. Tr.*).

Duchenne described bulbar paralysis.

Quain observed "tabby cat" fatty heart in anemia.

1852 Periarteritis nodosa described in *Rokitansky's* "Diseases of the Arteries" (Kussmaul, 1866).

1853 *A. King* gave name, "Chloroma" to green tumors (*Mo. J. M. Sc.*). (Balfour, 1834.)

Paget's "Surgical Pathology."

1853-54 *Falret's* cyclical (manic depressive) insanity (*Bull. Acad. de méd.*).

1854 *Remak* derived skin cancer from the epidermis, not from connective tissue. (*Hannover*, 1852; *Thiersch*, 1865; *Waldeyer*, 1872, adenocarcinoma.)

A. von Graefe elucidated nature of glaucoma, keratoconus.

1857 Philadelphia Pathological Society founded.

Pasteur's recognition of living ferments paved the way to the modern knowledge of bacterial causes of diseases (*Compt. Rend. Acad. d. sc.*).

1857-72 *Hebra* described many new skin diseases (lichen ruber, erythema multiforme, etc.).

1858 *Virchow's* "Cellularpathologie" published ("Omnis cellula e cellula").

1860 *Zenker* described trichinosis.

Samuel Gross described prostatorrhea (*Tr. Med. Soc. Penna.*).

1861 *Ménière* described special type of vertigo ("Ménière's disease").

Broca attributed aphasia to lesion of third left frontal convolution (*Bull. Soc. Anat.*).

Jonathan Hutchinson described "Heredito-Syphilitic Struma" and pegged teeth (B.M.J.)

1862 *Raynaud's* thesis "Sur l'asphyie locale et la gangrène symmetrique des extrémités."

William Little: cerebral diplegia from birth injury.

1863-67 *Virchow's* "Die krankhaften Geschwülsten."

1864 *Charcot* and *Robin* founded *J. de l'Anat. et de la Physiol. nor. et path.*

Zenker described degeneration of muscle ("Ueber die Veränderungen" etc., Leipzig).

Peacock's study of congenital anomalies of the heart.

1865 *Mendel's* observation on plant heredity (*Verh. Naturf. Ver. im Brunn*).

Villemin's "Cause et nature de la tuberculose" gave experimental proof of its infectiousness. (*Klencke,* 1843.)

1867 *Volkmann:* destructive uterine moles (chorionepithelioma). (*Marchand,* 1895.)

Golgi's description of psammoma (endothelioma) placed sarcoma on modern basis.

1868 *W. Meyer:* first adequate description of "adenoids" (*Hosp. Tid. Kjop.*). (*Czermak,* 1860.)

1871 *Weigert* studied smallpox and stained bacteria in tissues with carmine (coagulation necrosis). (*Centralbl. f. med. Wiss.*)

1871-72 *Gull* and *Sutton's* arterio-capillary fibrosis of chronic renal disease.

1872 *G. Huntington's* hereditary chorea (*Med. & Surg. Rep.,* Lyon, 1863).

A. Daae: Epidemic myalgia (Devil's grip). (*Finsen,* 1856; *Dabney,* 1888; *Sylvest,* 1934.)

1873 *Rustitzki* described multiple myeloma.

Cohnheim elucidated mechanism of inflammation and rôle of leukocytes. ("Neue Untersuchungen"). (See Wm. Addison's "Blood Corpuscles, Inflammation," 1843.)

Charcot differentiated amyotrophic lateral sclerosis.

1874 *Gull* described myxedema.

Paget's precancerous disease of the nipple (*St. Bart. Hosp. Rep.*).

Durante proposed embryonal cell theory of cancer origin. (*Cohnheim,* 1877; *Ribbert,* 1895.)

Kussmaul related fatal coma to diabetes *Deutsch. Arch. f. klin. Med.*).

Henoch: "A Peculiar Form of Purpura."

1875 *Lösch* associated amebae with a special type of dysentery.

William Pepper observed bone marrow changes in pernicious anemia (*Am. J. M. Sc.*). (*E. Neumann,* 1868, *Zbl. f. Med. Wiss.*)

Hughlings Jackon's unilateral type of epilepsy (*Brit. M. J.*).

1876-77 *Koch* and *Pasteur's* studies on anthrax inaugurated modern study of bacterial causes of disease (*Beitr. Biol. Pflanzen* and *Comp. rend. Acad. d. Sci.*).

Manson demonstrated rôle of insects as vectors of disease (Filaria by mosquitoes) (*Customs Gaz., Shanghai*).

1876 *Thomsen* described myotonia in his own person (Arch. f. Psych.).

Hanot described "Primary Biliary Hypertrophic Cirrhosis."

1877 *Paget's* osteitis deformans (*Med. Chir. Tr.*).

Bezold described mastoiditis, (*Arch. f. Ohrenh.*). (*Warnet,* 1873.)

Eck developed the "Eck fistula" for experimental study of liver diseases.

1877-80 *Cohnheim* transmitted tuberculosis experimentally by inoculation of rabbit's eye ("Vorlesungen").

1878 *Weir Mitchell* described erythromelalgia (*Am. J. M. Sc.*).

Abbé introduced oil immersion lens.

1878-79 *Erb* dèscribed myasthenia gravis (*Arch. f. Psych.*) . (*Goldflam*, 1891; *Oppenheim*, 1898.)

1879 *Ponfick* established pathology of human actinomycosis (*Berl. klin. Wchnschr.*) .

Psitticosis recognized as a disease of man (*Ritter* and *Eberth*) .

"Roger's disease": congenital defect of cardiac septum (*Bull. Acad. d. méd.*) .

1881 *Wernicke's* "Lehrbuch" described acute hemorrhagic poliencephalitis.

1882 *Koch's* discovery of tubercle bacillus (*Berl. klin. Wchnschr.*) .

Weigert described tuberculosis of veins and promulgated law of overgrowth of connective tissue in repair (*Arch. f. path. Anat.*) .

Golgi established principle of compensatory hypertrophy (and of regeneration of parenchyma, 1884) .

von Recklinghausen described neurofibromatosis (*Alexander,* 1800) ; also described carcinoids of the digestive tract.

Gaucher described lipoid splenomegaly ("De l'epithelioma primitif de la rate," Thesis, Paris) .

Quincke's angioneurotic edema (*Monatschr. f. prakt. Derm.*) .

1883 *Morvan* described syringomyelia (*Gaz. hebd. de méd.*) . (*Kahler,* 1882.)

Grawitz described renal tumors of adrenal origin (*Arch. f. path. Anat.*) .

Ebstein produced renal calculi experimentally (*Kong. f. inn. Med.*) .

1884 *Horsley* produced experimental myxedema by thyroidectomy (*Lancet*) .

Metchnikoff named "phagocytes" and demonstrated their importance in inflammation. (See *Allg. Wien med. Ztg.*, trans. from Russian.)

Flemming emphasized the rôle of the lymphocytes and lymphatics in inflammation.

Duhring described dermatitis herpetiformis (*J.
A. M. A.*).

1885 *Delafield* and *Prudden's* "Textbook of Pathology," first modern American textbook on the
subject.

1886 *Charcot-Marie-Tooth:* Peroneal type of muscular atrophy (*Rev. de méd.*).

Fitz named perforating appendicitis and established its importance (*Tr. A. Am. Phys.*).
(*Mestivier,* 1759; *Parkinson,* 1812.)

von Mering produced phlorhizin diabetes experimentally (*Kong. f. inn. Med.*).

Ziegler founded *Beiträge zur path. Anat. u.
Allgem. Path.*

Marie connected lesion of the pituitary with
acromegaly. (*Wilks,* 1869.)

Bard's "omnis cellula e cellula ejusdem generis."

Weil described infectious jaundice (*Deutsch.
Arch. f. klin. Med.*). (*Botkin,* 1889.)

Gee described coeliac disease. (*Herter,* 1918.)

Hirschsprung described congenital megacolon
(*J. f. Kinderh.*). (*Billard,* 1820.)

1887 *H. Sewell* discovered antitoxic form of resistance to disease (snake venom).

Lichtheim observed spinal cord changes in pernicious anemia (*Kong. f. inn. Med.*).

1888 *Dercum* described adiposis dolorosa (*U. of
Pennsylvania Med. Mag.*).

Fallot described the tetralogy of congenital
heart disease.

1889 *von Mering* and *Minkowski* removed pancreas
experimentally to cause diabetes (*Arch. f.
exper. Path. u. Pharm.*).

Hanau's successful transplantation of animal
tumors inaugurated experimental study of
cancer (*Fortschr. d. Med.*).

von Jaksch described pseudoleukemia of children (*Wien. klin. Wchnschr.*).

E. *Pfeiffer* observed glandular fever in children.

Reginald Harrison described a human cancer caused by a parasite (bilharzia) (*Lancet*).

Fitz described hemorrhagic necrosis of the pancreas.

1890   *Marie's* hypertrophic osteoarthropathy (*Rev. de méd.*). (*Bamberger*, 1889.)

1892   *Ivanowski* inaugurated study of viruses and of causes of plant diseases (mosaic disease of tobacco). (Foot and mouth disease, *Löffler and Frosch*, 1898.)

Woodhead founded *Journal of Pathology and Bacteriology.*

"*Mikulicz's* disease." (*Billroth* Festschrift.)

Vaquez described polycythemia vera (*Soc. de biol.*). (Osler, *Am. J. M. Sc.*, 1903.)

Milroy described hereditary edema of the legs.

1893   *Theobald Smith* and *Kilbourne* discovered intermediate host in Texas fever (tick).

1894   *Fournier* established "parasyphilitic" nature of paresis and tabes dorsalis.

Bruce showed rôle of tsetse fly in African sleeping sickness.

Guido Banti described splenomegaly with hepatic cirrhosis.

1895   *Kummel* described traumatic spondylitis (*Deutsch. med. Wchnschr.*).

Hand established syndrome of diabetes insipidus, bone defects, and exophthalmos. (*Schüller*, 1915; *Christian*, 1920.)

1897   *Mallory* and *Wright's* "Pathological Technique" published.

1898   *Hayem* described hemolytic ictero-anemia (*Presse méd.*). (*Chauffard, Minkowski*, 1900.)

Simond demonstrated transmission of plague by fleas (*Ann. Inst. Past.*).

N. Gwyn isolated paratyphoid fever. (*Achard* and *Bensaude*, 1896.)

Kraepelin introduced dementia praecox and other classes of psychoses ("Lehrbuch").

Foundation of the *Deutsche Pathologische Gesellschaft.*

1899 *Sternberg* established histology of Hodgkin's disease (*Centralbl. f. d. Grenzgeb.*). (*Reed,* 1902; *Longcope,* 1903.)

1900 *Reed, Carroll, Lazear* and *Agramonte* demonstrated transmission of yellow fever by mosquito. (*Finlay,* 1881.)

Dukes described "fourth disease." (*Filatow,* 1885.)

Danysz began experimental study of epidemics. (*Flexner, Webster,* 1918.)

Landsteiner's four blood groups explained transfusion hemolysis.

1901 *Opie* related islands of Langerhans to diabetes (*J. Exper. Med.*).

William Pepper, Jr. outlined syndrome of adrenal medullary tumors (*Am. J. M. Sc.*). (Hutchinson type, 1907, *Am. J. M. Sc.*)

American Association of Pathologists and Bacteriologists founded.

Fröhlich's "adiposo-genital dystrophy" of pituitary origin. (*Wien. klin. Runds.*)

Ayerza lectured on cardiacos negros, due to pulmonary artery sclerosis (Buenos Aires thesis, 1909).

1902 *Hansemann's* concept of anaplasia in cancer ("Die mikroskopische Diagnose").

Richet developed "anaphylaxis" and coined term.

1902-15 Pathologic physiology of heart mechanism established by *Mackenzie, Thomas Lewis,* and others.

1903   *Metchnikoff* successfully inoculated apes with syphilis (*Cong. Internat. d'hyg.*) .

      Arthus phenomenon (*Comp. rend. Soc. de biol.*) .

1905   *Schaudinn* and *Hoffmann* discovered Treponema pallidum (*Arb. a. d. Kais. Ges.*) .

1906   *Naunyn* introduced term "acidosis" as found in diabetes. (*Boussingault,* 1850.)

1906-08   Causation of heart block demonstrated experimentally (*Erlanger*) and clinically (*Stengel, Aschoff, Tawara* and others) .

      Barany: nystagmus test for vestibular disease.

1907   *Searcy* recognized endemicity of pellagra in U. S. A. (*Gray,* 1864.)

      Albrecht founded *Frankfurter Zeitschrift für Pathologie.*

1908   *Pathologica* founded by *Mario Segale.*

      MacCallum and *Voigtlin* demonstrated relation of tetany to calcium metabolism (*Johns Hopkins Hosp. Bull.*) .

1908-24   Nature of rickets demonstrated experimentally by *Findlay, MacCallum, Mellanby, Hess, Steenbock, et al.*

1909   *Nicolle* demonstrated experimental transmission of typhus by the louse (*Compt. rend. Acad. d. Sc.*) .

1910   Tissue cultures inaugurated by *R. G. Harrison's* growth of nerve cells in vitro (*J. Exper. Zool.*) .

      Libman's subacute bacterial endocarditis (*Am. J. M. Sc.*) . (Schottmüller's "E. Lenta"; *Osler,* 1885.)

      J. B. Herrick identified sickle cell anemia (*Arch. Int. Med.*) .

1911   *P. Rous* discovered filtrable sarcoma of fowls (*J. Exper. Med.*) .

      de Beurmann and *Gougerot* described sporotrichosis (*Arch. f. Derm. u. Syph.*) .

1912 *Kinnear Wilson's* lenticular nucleus degeneration with liver lesions (*Brain*).

Carrel demonstrated potential immortality of mammalian tissue (in vitro growth) (*J. Exper. Med.*).

1913 *Aschoff* and *Landau's* reticulo-endothelial system (*Sitz. Ver. z. Freiburg*).

Reschad and *Schilling Torgau* demonstrated monocytic leucemia.

Durant et al. described lymphogranuloma inguinale (climatic bubo).

American Society of Experimental Pathology founded.

Fibiger produced cancer experimentally by nematode action in rats' stomachs (*Berl. klin. Wchnschr.*).

Ramon y Cajal modernized study of gliomata. (*del Rio Hortega*, 1919.)

K. Faber: simple hypochromic anemia.

1913 *Maud Slye's* studies of cancer inheritance.

G. W. Whipple's experimental studies of anemia and of regeneration of blood proteins.

1914 *Niemann's* lipoid histiocytosis (Niemann-Pick's disease) (*Jahrb. f. Kinderh.*).

Simmonds' pituitary type of dwarfism (*Deutsch. path. Gesellsch.*).

Volhard and *Fahr's* "Die Brightsche Krankheit" established modern concept of Bright's Disease, based on the nature of the significant lesion.

1915 Trench fever observed in British and German Armies. (*Graham*, 1915; *Werner*, 1916).

1915-18 *L. Henderson, van Slyke et al.* established chemical constituents of blood and importance of acid-base equilibria.

1916 *Yamagiwa* and *Ichikawa* produced skin cancer experimentally with tar (*Mitt. d. med. Fak.*, Tokyo).

National Research Council organized at Washington.

1917 Bacteriophage described by *d'Herelle* (*Twort*, 1915).

Importance of constitutional disposition established by *J. Bauer*.

1918 *von Economo* discovered lethargic encephalitis (*Wien. klin. Wchnschr.*).

Frank established thrombocytopenic basis of purpura hemorrhagica (*Reichs. Med. Anz.*).

The suspension stability of the erythrocytes correlated with disease by *Fahreus* (Bioch. Zts.).

(See John Hunter's lectures, 1786.)

1920 *Ewing* distinguished "endothelial myeloma" of bone. (Arch. Surg., 1922.)

1921 Discovery of insulin by *Banting* and *Best* elucidated nature of diabetes (*J. Lab. & Clin. Med.*). (*Schaffer*, "The Endocrine Organs," 1916.)

Sampson's chocolate cysts of peritoneum (endometriosis).

1921- *Houssay:* Disturbed pituitary function, especially in relation to diabetes (*C. N. Long*, 1933).

1922 *Schultz* described agranulocytosis (*Deutsch. med. Wchnschr.*).

1925 *Wolbach* and *Howe* established histopathology of vitamin A deficiency (*J. Exper. Med.*).

Heidelberger, Avery and *Goebel* demonstrated that resistance to infection depends on chemical constitution of invading organism (*Neufeld*, 1910).

1926 *Minot* and *Murphy's* liver diet elucidated nature of pernicious anemia (*J. A. M. A.*).

1926-34 Hyperparathyroidism and relation to bone disease established by *Mandl, Collip, Barr, Albright et al.*

1927 *Cooley's* erythroblastosis of infants.

1929 *von Gierke's* glycogen disease of liver, kidneys and heart (*Beit. z. path. Anat.*).
1931 *Shope* demonstrated the combined action of a virus in swine influenza.
1932 *Cushings'* pituitary basophilism (*Bull. Johns Hopkins Hosp.*).
1934 *Collip's* concept of anti-hormones developed to resist hormonal action.
      Rowntree and *Clark* demonstrated the inherited rôle of the thymus in precocious growth.
      Goldblatt produced prolonged hypertension experimentally. (J. E. M.)
1935 A virus disease (mosaic tobacco disease) shown by *Stanley* to be due to a crystallizable protein. (*Science.*)

BIBLIOGRAPHY

CASTIGLIONI, A. Storia della Medicina. Ed. 2, Milan, 1936.
CHIARI, H. In: Neuburger and Pagel's Hand. d. Gesch.
    der Med., 2: 473, 1903 (especially useful for ref-
    erences to works of lesser known pathologists
    from the sixteenth century on).
DEZEIMERIS, O. Dictionnaire de la Medicine. Paris, 1828.
GARRISON, F. H. History of Medicine. Ed. 4, Phila., Saun-
    ders, 1929.
HIRSCH, A. Biographisches Lexikon (5 vols.). Vienna,
    Urban & Schwarzenberg, 1884-88; also 2 vols.
    "Neuzeit," 1932-33.
ISENSEE, E. Gesch. der Med. Berlin, 1840-45.
LONG, E. R. Selected Readings in Pathology. Springfield,
    Ill., Thomas, 1929.
MAJOR, R. H. Classic Descriptions of Disease. Springfield,
    Ill., Thomas, 1932.
MOODIE, R. Paleopathology. Urbana, Ill., Univ. Illinois
    Pr., 1923.
NEUBURGER, M. History of Medicine. Trans. by E. Play-
    fair, 1910 and 1925, incomplete.
NEUBURGER, M., and PAGEL, J. Hand. d. Gesch. der Med. (3
    vols.) Jena, Fischer, 1902-05, 2: 63.
PREUSS, J. Biblisch. Talmudische Med. Berlin, 1911.
RUFFER, S·R A. Studies in the Paleopathology of Egypt.
    Chicago, 1921.
SINGER, C. A Short History of Medicine. N. Y., 1928.
SMITH, E., and DAWSON, W. R. Egyptian Mummies. N. Y.,
    Dial, 1924.
SPRENGEL, K. P. J. Versuch einer prag. Geschichte d. Arz-
    neikunde, Halle, 1792.
SUDHOFF, K. "Klassiker" der Medizin, *Arch. f. Gesch. d.
    Med.*, Leipzig, 1927.
The Sydenham Society Publications, Old and New Series,
    London, 1859-1907 (give good translations of
    many of the classics mentioned in these pages).
THOMPSON, R. C. *Proc. Roy. Soc. Med., Sec. Med. Hist.*,
    17: 1, 1923-24, 19: 29, 1925-26.
WITHINGTON, E. T. Medical History from the Earliest
    Times. London, 1894.
WUNDERLICH, C. A. Geschichte der Medicin. Stuttgart,
    1859.

INDEX OF PERSONAL NAMES

INDEX OF SUBJECTS

197